Cindy, your book is so beautiful!!!! It is lovely to look at and I almost cried when I looked inside and began my reading. I am really impressed. I feel so happy that you have portrayed my dads work in such a nice way.... The book has a really nice feel to it too.
            Julietta St. John

Cindy has managed to put into words the very subtle and elusive quality of Metamorphosis. Some have sensed this elusive element during a treatment or even upon entering a room where Metamorphosis is being practiced. This book is such a valuable resource not only for understanding the substance of Metamorphosis but for experiencing its spirit as well.
            Nancy Stetson, a student of
            Robert St. John's for over 20 years.

I just wanted to tell you how terrific you are! Each time I go through it, I see how much you put into each sentence.
            Dr. Shoshana Savyon
            Jerusalem, Israel

This book is a theoretical exploration of how things really work. Very difficult to translate theory to it's application, but you've done a wonderful job with it.
            Mary Kopac, North Carolina

At last I have found a book that brings me closer to the substantial essence of Metamorphosis. Your book helped me to find and thus to give a clearer explanation about the principles of Metamorphosis, in such a way that I have found a renewed passion in the work. Thank you!
            Petra van Noort, New York

Your book is really great. It makes the principles very accessible. Clear, well organized and user friendly.
            Michael Edan, New York

I did not expect the book to be so good, as Metamorphosis is a hard subject to write about. The information is accessible without losing the essence and spirit of Metamorphosis. In fact, it is a very good demonstration of the balance of afference and efference. I was quite delighted by it!

Angie Lyndon, Australia

You have really enlightened me with this book about life in general and I can see my patterns and understand the questions I have always had but didn't know how to put them into words. Metamorphosis is more than I imagined...thanks.

P.T. Thompkins, Texas

I want to thank you for all the time and energy you put into writing this book, it was a pleasure to read!

Cindy Carmichael, Washington

Metamorphosis

Metamorphosis

Creating Consciousness Through Touch

Cindy Silverlock

KINI PUBLISHING

Santa Rosa, California, U.S.A

Metamorphosis: Creating Consciousness Through Touch
Kini Publishing
PO Box 2945
Santa Rosa, CA 95405

Illustrators: James Franklin Pierce, Jody Grovier and Catherine Greco
Interior Design: Lorien Fenton
Cover Design: Lorien Fenton and Cindy Silverlock
Photo: Rob Kunkle - http://goodlux.com

Published by: Kini Publishing
ISBN# 978-0-9722897-4-0
LCCN# 2005927111
Printed in the United States

Disclaimer: The Metamorphosis Center and Cindy Silverlock disclaim all
responsibility for any adverse effects that might occur as a result of the
application of any of the information contained in this book. Metamorphosis
is not to be used in lieu of appropriate medical care. Please contact a
physician or therapist if you have any concerns regarding your health.

Acknowledgments

Time spent in conversation with Robert St. John over the years had a tremendous impact on every aspect of my life. Robert was Metamorphosis; its essence was within him.

By living the work, Robert showed me that to teach means to introduce the principles, guiding people to a place where they can experience them on their own. Robert's humility taught me that no one is an authority on healing or life. He encouraged strength and independent thinking in others.

Robert's tremendous ability to see into the patterns of life and also find humor in them was a tremendous gift. He did not pretend to be an ideal person, which imparted an acceptance of our individual and collective short-comings. At the same time he created a simple approach to self-healing allowing us to become what we strive to be.

A heartfelt thank you to Nancy Stetson for reading this book in many stages of revision. Nancy's genuine interest in it helped me move through the various challenges I experienced during the writing process. Her affection for Metamorphosis and Robert were evident.

I want to acknowledge Lynn Hatswell for her lecture on afference and efference, and how they influence our personalities and relationships. Her lecture was helpful in grounding these principles into everyday thinking.

A special thank you to my husband Dean for being an endless source of support. Recognizing patterns within oneself and in a relationship is both challenging and exciting. I am thankful to have such a special and loving partner to do this with.

—Cindy Silverlock

Foreword

Written by Nancy Stetson

When I met Robert St. John in 1976, his thinking was revolutionary. To acknowledge that thought creates reality and to begin with thought in the creation of a healing system was such a relief to me. It is mind that creates and mind that heals, thus the effectiveness of different healing modalities that have contradictory designations for the same points. Robert always said that the reflex points he discovered were accurate to the best of his knowledge, but at the same time it was his act of creation that set the structure in place and enabled it to work. It is the intent of the practitioner that brings results and the structure of the therapy is the means to focus that intent.

Paralleling this revelation was the knowledge that one could access a time period, even the time before conception through the simple tool that Robert provided. He found that he could access that timeline through the spinal reflex points on the feet, head and hands. Metamorphosis opened up a whole new world of possibilities to me. During the next twenty years I spent as much time as I could with Robert as he continued to explore and develop his work.

Cindy has done an excellent job of conveying the principles of Metamorphosis. This is not easy to do for many reasons. Some people would like Metamorphosis to be made into a technique which they could simply follow. This would be contradictory to the essence of Metamorphosis. Others would like scientific proof. Robert's attitude was that it is counterproductive to test people, then label them and look for particular results. He refused to do that even if it interfered with his ability to get the work accepted. Labeling people fixes them in that condition as thought is so powerful.

We have been told that we must look outside of ourselves to know what is true. The power of an agreed upon reality is so strong that it is hard to get people to trust themselves. But now even science has come to the limits of its ability to fix and define material reality. The influence of thought on the results of any experiment, whether in psychology or physics, is increasingly becoming a point of focus. Robert always encouraged people to connect to their own innate intelligence. The shift to the point of view of consciousness and creativity is what Metamorphosis is all about.

Since 1962 Robert saw a number of changes in the relationship of afference (consciousness) and efference (action). Whereas efference had been dominant, which explains the rise of science, it is now at the service of afference. There is much confusion as the old forms try to hold on, but we are moving into a time of inner knowing. Robert saw Metamorphosis as a means of helping people make this transition. When there is a balance of afference and efference, awareness moves spontaneously into action with no blocks. This is the goal of Metamorphosis, to be in the present moment.

Reading this book has been a delight for me. Cindy has managed to put into words the very subtle and elusive quality of Metamorphosis.

Some have sensed this elusive element during a treatment or even upon entering a room where Metamorphosis is being practiced. This book is such a valuable resource not only for understanding the substance of Metamorphosis but for experiencing its spirit as well.

Contents

In Appreciation

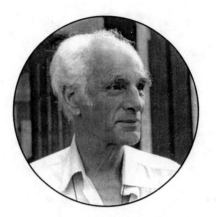

ROBERT ST. JOHN
1914 - 1996

Metamorphosis is my passion and it is with pleasure that I share this work with you. The information presented in this book comes from my understanding based on eighteen years of practicing, teaching and contemplating Metamorphosis.

Introduction

Metamorphosis is about creating your life

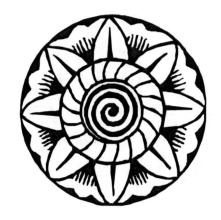

Metamorphosis is a self-healing art and a philosophy on creating greater consciousness within. We use the concept of reflex points to address the unconscious blocks that create conflict, disease and disharmony in our lives and in our collective experience. As we change, the world around us changes.

As these patterns release we experience greater awareness or enhanced intuition, better health, genuine relationships and less conflict in life. Metamorphosis is simple to use, easy to learn and can be used as part of your daily life. You can work on yourself, others and animals.

This book is written as a guide to Metamorphosis. My intent is to introduce the principles and practice of Metamorphosis, allowing you to find and experience its essence for yourself. I hope to inspire you to feel that you can grasp Metamorphosis and begin to practice it in your own home. It is a wonderful feeling to know that you have the ability and means to increase your intuitive awareness and improve the quality of life for yourself and your family. You do not need to have any previous experience to understand or practice Metamorphosis. An open mind and patience are all that you need.

I introduce the principles throughout this book, encouraging you to stop and think about what is being said as you read. I also repeat a few essential ideas throughout the text. Most likely you will find it helpful to read the book several times, letting the information sink in over time.

The essence of Metamorphosis comes from its principles. While there is a hands-on application, or practice, with Metamorphosis, it is the principles that are most important. As you begin to consider the principles, as well as the nature of creation, healing and life in general, your perspectives and possibly your life may start to change.

In order to practice Metamorphosis, all you need is an understanding of the essence of the philosophy, or the gist of it, without being overly concerned with the details or data. While Metamorphosis is practical and simple, it is not linear. At first, it may seem like a huge body of abstract or 'way out' concepts.

The journey of looking at the nature of patterns and conditioned thinking within yourself and the world can make the philosophy seem a little overwhelming at times. This is actually a good thing, because it means that you are beginning to truly think for yourself, realizing that reality is based on perceptions, which are primarily determined by your underlying stress patterns. As you consider the principles and practice the work, the simplicity of Metamorphosis becomes more apparent.

Metamorphosis is an intuitive approach and is not a technique. Robert did use the term technique in his first two books, but he later said that the nature of the word was not appropriate. A technique implies that you follow a set way of doing something, which can be replicated. Metamorphosis is about tuning-in and using your intuition, which cannot be replicated.

Consider the difference between traveling by tour bus and traveling on your own. Traveling by tour bus takes you to pre-determined sites, which you are guided to and can visit on a limited time schedule. You will probably benefit from and enjoy the experience.

Traveling on your own requires you to rely on and think for yourself. You have to take the time to get to know the country, city or terrain you are visiting. You may need to inquire about where the locations are that you want to visit or you may just happen upon them, which is even more exciting. The difference is that you really get to know the essence of the place where you are traveling. The experience becomes a part of you, rather than a memorable guided tour of the local tourist spots.

With Metamorphosis, you are your own tour guide. You have to take the time to get to know the principles, so that you will know the work from within. In doing this, Metamorphosis becomes a part of who you are. When you give a treatment, you bring this inner understanding to the treatment, rather than practicing from technique. This is the profundity of the work.

Metamorphosis is 'alive' which means it loses something when you try to explain it. Words help to communicate this subtle philosophy but they also get in the way. Keep in mind that Metamorphosis is not a treatment, you are not treating a person or symptom. (Some people use the word session instead of treatment.) The word work or working is not accurate either, as it implies effort. Words such as levels, shifting and process tend to portray a concept and yet are also not quite accurate. You get the idea!

Keep in mind as you read that the word healing is used throughout this book to mean creating awareness as well as a healthier and more harmonious approach to life. In doing this we cease to create illness, disharmony and conflict. It is important to recognize the distinction between ceasing to create and curing. We address underlying patterns of stress and therefore we cease to create stressful reactions to life. This is different than addressing symptoms and curing. This is really important in understanding the entire theme of Metamorphosis.

Metamorphosis introduces some unique ideas and may invite you to reconsider existing thoughts on creation, life, relationships and healing. Considering new possibilities can challenge existing paradigms and individual beliefs, which in turn often challenges your sense of reality and/or identity. When dealing with a concept that seems hard to believe or challenging, it is helpful to keep the idea in mind, rather than making one way right, which has to make all others wrong.

You may find it interesting and insightful to consider how your personal beliefs have shaped your reality. Take notice of how your perceptions change as you let go of your underlying stress patterns.

In an effort to understand Metamorphosis, people often try to compare it to approaches they are already familiar with. Although Metamorphosis may sound similar to other approaches, upon closer examination, it usually is not. It is helpful if you contrast Metamorphosis to other approaches, rather than compare them. In other words, it is helpful to notice the differences rather than the similarities.

If you decide that this point of view is fascinating, resonates with you or makes your life easier, I encourage you to observe the principles within your daily life.

Please note that in this book I discuss the principles before the practice. The principles create the intent for the practice. The second half of the book teaches you the practice of the work: working on the feet, hands, head and spine as well as working with the hand symbols.

Keep in mind as you read that it is more important that you connect with the spirit of the work than it is to remember data.

The History

As we change, the world around us changes

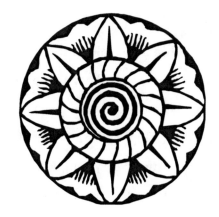

Originally called Prenatal Therapy, this body of work evolved into what is now known as Metamorphosis. Robert St. John began creating this work in England during the late 1950's. I use the word create rather than founded because I think the work developed out of his tremendous creativity.

While other people have had similar insights into the human dynamic and dilemmas, few have developed a way out. Not only did Robert find a way out, he created a simple, practical approach that anyone can learn to use in their daily life.

Robert was inspired to develop his own work based on several things he observed in his experience with the healing arts. While working with Naturopathic Medicine, Robert recognized that the focus of most healing approaches is on treating symptoms. While the symptoms usually went away after treatment, they often returned, or people experienced new symptoms, because the underlying patterns of stress causing the symptoms were not addressed.

The concept of Reflexology was an inspiration to Robert. For those of you not familiar with Reflexology, it is a system of working with reflex points on the feet, hands and sometimes the ears. The reflex points correspond with a map of the physical body.

Robert noticed that within Reflexology there were many maps of the feet, all a little different, yet they all worked. This observation suggested that reflex points can act as symbols for the intent given to them. The use of reflex points became the basis for developing the practice of Metamorphosis.

While working with the Bates Eye System, Robert discovered the principles of what he would later call afference and efference. It was his observation that people's primary attitude toward life was reflected in their eyesight. The shape of the eyeballs and the quality of vision expressed a chronic, compulsive attitude of mind. Those who tended to pull away from life often developed retreative eyesight, creating far-sightedness or hypermetropia, causing their eyeballs to sit slightly inward. This he termed afferent. Those who tended to push forward into life often developed near-sightedness or myopia, causing their eyeballs to sit slightly forward. This he termed efferent. These observations became the basis for the philosophy of Metamorphosis.

In considering the history of humanity, Robert noticed that the overall patterns of humanity have never really changed. Illness, disharmony, conflict and war have always been in existence. He realized that these primary stress patterns of humanity continue on because they have not been addressed at their origins. Throughout time we have focused primarily on symptoms rather than the cause behind the symptoms.

In observing the principles of life, Robert saw that the cause of all symptoms of disease and disharmony stem from what he called the separation of afference and efference. This separation caused oneness to become duality.

The cosmic phenomena he observed as the separation of afference and efference resulted in the creation of time, space, our universe and all life on earth. The separation was the onset of humanity's tensions, becoming the initial stress pattern for humanity and the primary source behind all of our personal and global dilemmas. The negative stress patterns are kept alive because they are passed on via genetic and karmic patterns. This means that stress can move through time and continue to influence each generation. These patterns become a part of our cellular makeup at conception. We are influenced by these patterns at conception and throughout our prenatal development as well as throughout life. The quality of our health and every aspect of our lives are influenced by these patterns.

Robert used the terms afference and efference as analogies or symbols to explain the dynamic of life on this planet. What he has done with his observations is create a unique perspective on creation and healing.

As Robert was making all of these observations, the practice of Metamorphosis began to reveal itself to him. As he practiced Reflexology, he began to notice that when he worked on people's heels they often spoke of troubles with their mothers. He began to see a pattern and wondered where the father was represented on the foot.

One morning while sitting in the bath, which is where Robert often gained insight, he saw the prenatal pattern in relationship to the feet. If the heel was the mother principle, birth, then it was only logical that conception was the father principle, as that is where his influence is introduced. He saw the conception point corresponded with an area on the big toe.

At this time he concluded that the reflex points for the spine represent the period of time between conception and birth. Robert was getting a grand picture of how to address the individual and collective disturbances that humanity and all life forms are subject to.

Understanding that reflex points act as symbols to communicate a given intent and recognizing that the spine is the central point of the body, Robert began to work on the feet from a different perspective than Reflexology. He began to consider the primary imbalance of humanity as a whole. His observations on what he termed afference and efference became the basis for this approach. As his perspective changed, his clients began to change on all levels, not just the physical. This was the beginning of Metamorphosis.

Despite the grandiose nature of the philosophy, Metamorphosis remains a simple and practical approach to address underlying stress patterns. The profundity lies in that we do not involve the intellect. We communicate the intention of Metamorphosis via reflex points directly to the unconscious mind—life force—cellular intelligence. The unconscious mind communicates with symbols, which is why it responds to this non-verbal approach.

Metamorphosis acknowledges that we are self-healing. Metamorphosis also recognizes that the primary principle of healing is intention. The scope of the intention is the key, for if your intent is to heal at the physical level, then that is the outcome. If your intent is to heal at the primary source of humanity's tensions, then that is the outcome. We are limited by the scope of our intention and what we believe can happen. Collectively, we are conditioned to believe that we need to rely on experts for our well-being. We often cannot fathom that we are capable of such tremendous change on our own.

Robert did a wonderful job of reminding us that we are innately self-healing, and when we step into that mind-set, our bodies and minds are capable of tremendous change—a true Metamorphosis.

The Principles

Metamorphosis means transmutation to a finer substance

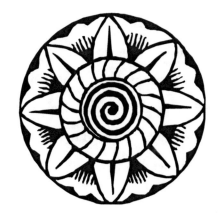

The principles of Metamorphosis are the essence of the work. The practice of Metamorphosis does not define the work; it offers a means to impart the principles.

Robert once explained to me that he needed to look at the theme of Metamorphosis in detail, in order to create the symbols for us to use. He said that he "set the work in the cosmos," so to speak, which enables us to work with the theme without having to intellectually understand the entire picture.

Robert also said that the information is the blueprint for the work, which gives you the basis from which to work. Once you embody the primary principles, the data is no longer necessary. The theme becomes inherent in your decision to practice Metamorphosis.

The primary principles of Metamorphosis are afference and efference and the prenatal pattern. The theme of afference and efference explains why humanity has its dilemmas and offers a new perspective on the dynamics of life, healing and relationships. The prenatal pattern offers a means to do something about our dilemmas.

It is helpful to realize that you do not need to fully understand the principles in order to practice Metamorphosis. The idea is not to study the theme but rather to experience it. Having an awareness of the principles 'activates' them, so to speak. Metamorphosis is a living theme which we naturally engage in whenever we practice the work as well as when we read, talk, or think about it. Keep in mind as you read that Metamorphosis is not linear. The information will weave together as a whole, creating a theme rather than a set of principles.

Afference & Efference

Because the concept of afference and efference is one of the primary principles of Metamorphosis, I will begin with a brief explanation of what they mean. At the end of this section I go into greater detail as to how their dynamic affects us in our daily lives.

Keep in mind that while all the principles work together, the theme of afference and efference bind everything together. While they appear to be an elusive concept at times, their meaning will begin to fall into place.

Robert observed that the dynamic of existence on this planet is based on what he termed afference and efference. Their interactive dynamic affects our health, personalities, relationships and global well-being, as well as influencing our views on life, creation, religion and healing.

The term afference defines the principles of consciousness and aware-ness, and the term efference defines the principles of action and response. Together they define the dynamic of all interactions within, interpersonally and globally, creating life as we know it. Afference is life itself and efference houses that life. Efference is the body and brain. The mind is the dual func-tion of afference and efference.

Afference and efference always operate together in a positive or negative manner. Similar to dancing, sometimes the dance flows and feels wonderful and sometimes it feels awkward or uncomfortable.

Afferent and efferent are Latin words that depict the movement inward and outward, respectively. In Metamorphosis they define the two primary attitudes of mind, depicting the compulsive nature to retreat from life or push forward into life.

People often try to equate afferent with introversion or yin and efferent with extroversion or yang. Although there are similarities, the overall picture is different. Relating afference and efference to another theory pulls in another school of thought, which, more often than not, takes you in a direc-tion other than the theme of Metamorphosis.

BLOCKS

We compulsively and unconsciously function from our blocks until they no longer exist. The practice of Metamorphosis is a letting go of these blocks.

Blocks are the unconscious stresses that interrupt or inhibit the natural flow of our life force. When the flow is interrupted it causes us to react to life, creating disturbance and disharmony in all levels of function. When we are in a reasonable balance of afference and efference we respond to life, which is a harmonious interaction with life and all living things.

A reaction is a stressed interaction with life and is expressed as disease, conditions, injury, disharmony and conflict. These can be experienced individually as well as collectively.

When our life force encounters a block it automatically expresses itself in a stressed manner. We use the word compulsion because this dynamic occurs without choice. Sometimes we are aware of these blocks that create our disturbances. Other times we cannot see that the disturbances in our lives come from within.

Robert referred to blocks of an afferent nature as karmic, meaning of the past, and existing in the realm of thought. (The word karmic is not to be confused with the Hindu use of the word.) They are expressed in relation to the head as mental tension, disturbance or illness.

Efferent blocks are genetic and passed on via maternal and paternal genes, tracing back to the beginning of your lineage. They are expressed physically, emotionally and behaviorally.

When in balance, you are living in the present moment. On occasion you get a glimpse of this balanced state when you are thoroughly engaging in something you enjoy. This is when everything comes together perfectly without effort, you are fully in the moment.

PATTERNS

Often referred to as underlying patterns or stress patterns, we use this term to explain the nature and expression of a block. Patterns can be expressed physically, mentally, emotionally, behaviorally and spiritually.

People experience physical patterns of pain, discomfort, injury and illness. Some people have emotions they regularly experience. This emotion is compulsive and the person often feels out of control and unable to respond in a desired or positive manner. They may regularly feel angry, frustrated, jealous, insecure or depressed. Mental patterns express themselves as mental illness, excessive worrying, anxiety and headaches. Sometimes it feels as if the mind won't shut off, keeping people awake at night.

Children often express compulsive behavior that stems from internal stress. I find it fascinating to observe children because you can often see patterns in their behavior and in their facial expressions. They are not trained to try and hide their patterns, as most adults are, so their patterns are often more apparent.

Spiritual patterns are often experienced as not feeling connected to a purpose in life. We are naturally connected to a greater consciousness but do not always realize it because our blocks create a sense of isolation or separation from source.

Addiction is a pattern of using something outside of yourself to cope with internal tension. Some patterns are expressed as attitudes such as poverty, survival, struggle or conflict. Many people's lives are filled with patterns of drama and chaos. We all have predominant patterns from which we compulsively and repeatedly function. These patterns tend to individually and collectively define our lives in subtle and significant ways.

Without judgment, begin to notice the patterns operating within yourself and others. You can usually see the patterns in others more easily than you can in yourself. You may start to realize that what you once thought was a personality trait is actually a pattern. You may also begin to feel more compassion for yourself and others as you notice the compulsive nature of your own patterns. Even better, you may realize that you can change these patterns.

When in a pattern, there are no options. The compulsive pattern kicks in automatically. Some people refer to this as having their "buttons pushed." We call it having your patterns stimulated.

As you let go of the blocks creating the patterns, you become less compulsive and reactive. You can begin to create your life rather than have your life created by your blocks and patterns.

We often feel the need to analyze our patterns in order to understand and change them. The practice of Metamorphosis addresses the primary source of our patterns: the tension between the imbalance of afference and efference. This allows for change without analysis.

TUNING-IN

Tuning-in simply means paying attention with an intuitive or inner awareness. When practicing Metamorphosis we tune-in to a reflex point without diagnosis or interpretation. Metamorphosis is non-verbal and non-directive.

As a practitioner, you are simply a catalyst. Paying attention to a reflex point, with the inherent intention of Metamorphosis, elicits a response from the innate intelligence of the person receiving the treatment. Consciousness is 'brought' to the unconscious patterns within, creating change at a cellular level.

Tuning-in is simply being present with another person and allowing healing or change to take place. This is the opposite of trying to direct or elicit change or healing. (Just a reminder, I use the word healing to mean creating a healthier and more harmonious approach to life.)

Tuning-in is a natural ability, some are just more aware of it than others. We have all experienced a time when we entered a room and sensed that an argument took place, simply because we are aware of tension in the air. Tuning-in to a reflex point is similar. When we practice Metamorphosis we become aware of the underlying tensions within that person. Like the argument, we do not necessarily know what the tension is about, but we are aware of it.

You can apply the concept of tuning-in throughout your daily life. Tune-in to the nature of the patterns operating within any personal or global interaction. This is how you will start to see the relationship of afference and efference all around you.

Tuning-in on a regular basis refines your intuition. You will begin to know things, because you are tuning-in to the patterns operating around you. Natural psychic awareness occurs without even trying; this is a natural result of your blocks clearing away.

IDENTIFICATION

Identification means to relate to or identify with.

We can all remember a time when we watched a movie or read a book and felt emotional. The emotional feeling goes away in a short time, once we stop identifying with the story or character.

While practicing Metamorphosis, we can feel the nature of a block, such as heat, cold, or exhaustion, for example, because we are identifying with it. It is helpful to notice any tendency to over-identify or under-identify with a person's patterns. When we over-identify we can become affected by another's condition. When we under-identify we remain totally detached. The ability to tune-in is lost and leads to working from technique.

Tuning-in is essential to knowing where to work and for how long. When you have a reasonable balance of afference and efference the ability to tune-in and identify is natural and does not lead to over or under-identification.

We also tend to identify with our own patterns, such as an illness or condition. People often say "I am" or "I have" such and such. Robert had a relative who appeared to have the symptoms of Down Syndrome at birth. Rather than label her as such, they practiced Metamorphosis on her and she developed into a girl without any symptoms of Down Syndrome. Robert's thinking was that it is better not to label anyone with an illness or condition so that they do not begin to identify with the pattern.

Let me share a story about my husband Dean. While his situation is of a lighter nature, the identification with a pattern is evident. Several years ago Dean began to experience trouble with his ankles. At that time he was not inclined toward Metamorphosis so I chose to observe his situation. A chiropractor told him that he had tendonitis, something he would have for the rest of his life. Dean was instructed to do stretching exercises every evening and ice the tendon regularly. He began to routinely sit in the recliner with an ice bag and do his stretches every evening.

What was interesting to observe was the incredible decline Dean experienced. Because golf is his passion, he envisioned that this would disable him from the game. As he further identified with his 'condition,' he began to lose his motivation in life and went into a depressive state.

Eventually Dean requested several Metamorphosis treatments. Within a short time he stopped using the ice bag. The choice was not a conscious one; it was as if he forgot all about his ankles. The problem simply went away, and it was such a subtle transition, that he did not even notice.

Dean's story is a perfect example of what can happen when we begin to identify with a symptom or situation as well as how easily we can move beyond the symptom when we decide to address the underlying pattern.

MOTIVE

Motive is a primary element in all of our thoughts and actions.

Motive is an important aspect of Metamorphosis. Without judgment, begin to notice your motives when you practice Metamorphosis on others. When you give a treatment, do you tend to take the role of the healer? Do you want people to regard you as a healer? Do you need people to change, such as a family member or spouse? Are you putting your own needs into the treatment, such as hoping for credit as the healer, repeat business or a referral? Of course we all experience these kinds of thoughts from time to time, but are they a primary motive? If so, it may be helpful to work on yourself.

As with all the principles of Metamorphosis, you can apply the concept of motive to your daily life. Notice the underlying motives operating within yourself and others throughout the day. Often someone's actions are not desirable, due to their underlying patterns, but their intent or motive is good. Sometimes a person's actions are desirable but their motive is self-serving, thus the ulterior motive. What motivates a person is often of more significance than their actions.

I find it helpful when dealing with people to notice their general nature instead of the negative aspects of their patterns. People tend to be either interested in what is good for the whole, or what is good for the self. Of course, a person's overall nature can change as they come into better balance.

INTENTION

Intention is the essence of healing.

Intention is of utmost importance because it non-verbally communicates your overall aim and determines the outcome of the treatment. Intention is vague unless you define it. The purpose of this book is to clarify the intent of Metamorphosis. The intent becomes inherent in your decision to give a Metamorphosis treatment. You do not need to think about the principles or intent prior to, or during, a treatment.

Consider the scope of the intention. Where does the intention lead to: a symptom, a period of time, or the underlying pattern behind the symptom or trauma? The scope of your intent determines the scope of the outcome. This is actually my own terminology to explain what Robert talked about, as I find it easy to get the point across using these words.

Robert noticed that when the intent was to heal a symptom, the symptom often went away. But because the underlying pattern was not addressed, the symptom returned or new ones often emerged. The person was then in a continual cycle of treating symptoms.

Throughout history, the desire to heal symptoms has resulted in an array of healing approaches, most of them limited in their scope of intention. Some modalities treat physical symptoms, others mental, emotional or behavioral. Some try to incorporate the symptoms of the whole person, but the focus is still on symptoms. This makes healing quite complicated and requires a hierarchy of experts.

Consider the scope of intention in relationship to an event or period of time. Are you looking back to childhood, birth, conception or a past life? The scope of the intention for Metamorphosis goes back to the origin of stress for humanity, the separation of afference and efference, which resulted in the creation of time and all the disturbances humanity struggles with. To focus on an event in time is a symptomatic approach. We are more interested in the underlying patterns of the past that continue to cause disturbance in the present. We are addressing the negative effects and influence of time.

As you let go of the negative influences of the past you do not need to re-enter, remember, or understand a previous stress or trauma. Focusing on stress from the past actually gets in the way of letting it go. The more you focus on a pattern or problem the less room it has to go away.

For those of you who like to understand the why's and how's of things, see if you can let go and allow insight to come to you. This is a natural process and does not require effort on your part. Allowing versus doing is a theme in Metamorphosis.

THE USE OF STRUCTURE

The use of structure is interesting to consider, for it affects us in ways that we may not notice.

It is important to realize that the practice of Metamorphosis is simply a structure that offers a means to impart the overall theme. If you can start to see the use of structure within any healing art and in the world around you, it dramatically changes your perspective and makes it easier to see the nature of the world around you.

Metamorphosis uses the structure of the prenatal pattern, explained in a moment, and the theme of afference and efference. The theme of afference and efference offers a perspective on creation, the onset of humanity's stress patterns and relationship dynamics. The use of reflex points and the prenatal pattern offer a structure to access these stress patterns.

The reduction of structure in the practice of Metamorphosis is a natural occurrence as we come closer to the balance of afference and efference. When you are functioning from a balance of afference and efference, you will naturally use the least amount of structure needed for the task at hand. Keep this in mind as you read this book, noticing the different levels of structure in the practice of Metamorphosis. As Robert engaged with the principles of Metamorphosis, his approach became more refined and more abstract. It was his thinking that the more abstract your approach, the more fundamental the level of change.

Consider the use of structure on a larger scale. Negative efference compulsively expands and adds unnecessary structure. Look at any large corporation or governing body; its endless structure often minimizes its effectiveness, and actually gets in the way of serving its purpose. It is easy to see the lack of consciousness (afference) in these structures.

Consider the nature of structure in relationship to the healing arts in general. A body of work may have started out as a simple approach, such as Metamorphosis, with a strong core essence to the work. Over time, as more and more efferently-oriented people get involved, technique, levels and/or hierarchy are often added or created. Generally, this kind of structuring adds more data and gets further away from the essence or nature of healing.

Hierarchy is a structure based on levels of importance and is abundant in the healing arts. There are those that are revered as, or deem themselves to be, healers or experts. The system of certification is also of this pattern for you could not certify another unless you considered yourself to be an authority. This is the reason that Robert did not create a certification program. He encouraged people to find the answers for themselves, and thus move away from the structure of hierarchy.

THE PRENATAL PATTERN

The prenatal pattern is a series of reflex points which act as symbols for the gestation period, the formative period from pre-conception to birth. The prenatal pattern offers a structure which enables us to address the primary stress patterns of humanity.

These primary stress patterns affect us individually based on the degree of genetic and karmic stress brought in at conception. Our underlying patterns are the primary stresses from which we consciously and unconsciously function. They determine what experiences are considered to be traumatic, based on how we perceive and handle the situations. Sometimes difficult situations make us stronger, and sometimes they continue to disturb us for years or throughout our lives.

This answers the frequently asked question of 'nature versus nurture.' Our womb and childhood environments are considered secondary stressors, for it is our underlying attitudes of mind that determines how we perceive and cope with these environments. These attitudes are what create our nature.

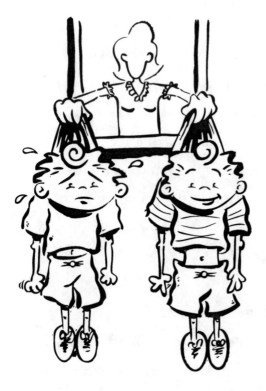

The following analogy, created by a Metamorphosis teacher in Australia, offers a picture of how our underlying attitudes of mind affect how we perceive life.

A mother of twin four-year-old boys is preparing scones for her friends, who are due to arrive. She realizes that she is out of eggs and running short on time, so she asks the boys to sit tight while she runs to the store.

While she is out, they decide to help, getting flour all over the counters and floor. Their mother, seeing this upon her return, is livid. In her frustration, she grabs the boys by their shirt collars and hangs them out the window, shakes them a bit, and brings them back in.

Thirty years later, one of the boys is a pilot, loves strong women and Danish pastries. The other one is afraid of heights, hates domineering women and is allergic to white flour products. During therapy, he remembers that at four years old his mother tried to kill him.

Each boy perceived the situation based on his underlying patterns or attitudes of mind. These underlying, unconscious attitudes are behind our individual and collective disturbances and determine what we experience as traumatic.

When we experience unconscious, internal stress, we find it harder to cope with external stress. The degree of internal stress is due to our underlying patterns.

This perspective gives us the realization that we cannot blame our womb or birth experience, childhood or parents as much as we might like to. Robert had a saying, "just get on with it," meaning focus on the present rather than the past. He also used to say, "just get on with the washing up." In other words, do you inspect and analyze every piece of food on your dirty dishes or do you just wash them? Something to think about!

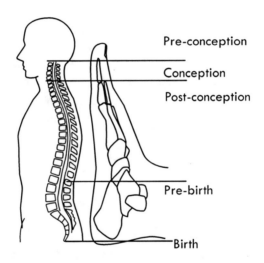

Pre-conception

Conception

Post-conception

Pre-birth

Birth

The Prenatal Pattern ©
*This diagram gives you a visual of the prenatal pattern
in relation to the feet and spine.*

Pre-conception

Pre-conception is the period prior to physical manifestation; it is the gathering of all your karmic influences. Karmic, in this sense, means in the realm of thought and of the past.

Pre-conception is registered within the pineal, pituitary and conception points.

Physically, pre-conception affects the sinuses and head from the area above the jaw line.

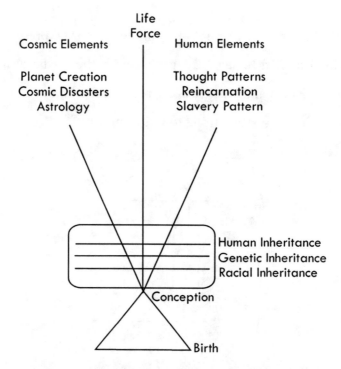

Life
Force

Cosmic Elements   Human Elements

Planet Creation   Thought Patterns
Cosmic Disasters   Reincarnation
Astrology   Slavery Pattern

Human Inheritance
Genetic Inheritance
Racial Inheritance

Conception

Birth

Pre-conception Diagram ©
This diagram gives you a visual of the overall theme.
This is a simplified re-creation of the diagram in Robert St. John's
"Metamorphosis a Text Book on Prenatal Therapy."

The pre-conception diagram offers a means to visualize the collective and individual influences that can enter at conception. Everything above the triangle represents the karmic patterns, the non-physical patterns that exist in the form of thought. The tip of the triangle represents conception, the moment when the influences that pertain to that individual, their genetic and karmic patterns, enter into physical form. The triangle represents the gestation period from conception to birth.

This diagram presents the theme of what we are working with in the practice of Metamorphosis. We address these underlying stress patterns via the spinal reflex points on the feet, hands and head, as well as when working directly on the spine, or when using the hand symbols.

The cosmic elements refer to the patterns of our planet and universe that have had an effect on all forms of life since the beginning of creation, including the separation of afference and efference.

The human elements refer to the patterns of humanity as a whole, from the beginning of human existence.

Astrology is based on the alignment of the planets at the exact time of our birth and the influence they have on us. The idea with Metamorphosis is that as we come into better balance we are less negatively influenced by things outside of ourselves, including the planets. This means that we can transcend our astrological charts.

Reincarnation is the concept that people live many lives. Robert said that a recollection of past lives does not necessarily mean we lived those lives, but possibly, when people die their unresolved thought patterns reside in time and space. During pre-conception, if a person has an affinity with a pattern of thought from a previous life, it may become a karmic pattern and have an influence on their life.

Whether reincarnation exists isn't really the point. The idea is to consider how collectively we tend to get attached to particular ways of thinking, which creates belief systems. More importantly, what we are concerned with is that something of the past is influencing us in the present, which to some extent means we are 'stuck' in the past. The aim of Metamorphosis is to let go of the negative influences of the past.

The slavery pattern has always had an influence on humanity. Throughout history mankind has enslaved groups of people and continues to enslave animals for entertainment and as beasts of burden. The mindset of using labor as a workforce, the working class, is also of this pattern.

The human inheritance refers to the patterns unique to mankind. Keep in mind that the disturbances of the negative afferent-efferent pattern affect all life on this planet.

The genetic inheritance refers to the patterns within your particular lineage, back to your origins, which are passed on via the maternal and paternal genes.

The racial inheritance refers to thought patterns in relation to your particular race or culture, back to its origin. Each race and culture has its own unique history and patterns.

All of these influences are a result of the separation of afference and efference. Their influence on humanity and each individual is primarily unconscious, which is why we often cannot find the cause of our individual and collective disturbances. When we limit the scope of our intention we limit our ability to create and heal. Going back to the origin of all the patterns affecting humanity means that we encompass all aspects of our patterns and not just the aspects we can intellectually comprehend or interpret.

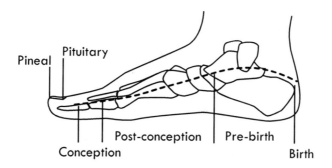

The pineal and pituitary reflex points represent the principle of life, that which manifests outside of the physical realm. The pineal reflex is located on the upper, inner edge of the big toenail. The pineal represents the absolute principle of life. The pituitary reflex point is the bottom of the inner edge of the big toenail. The pituitary represents the principle of life that is comprehensible to the human mind.

Conception

Conception is the moment in time when all your genetic and karmic influences enter into physical form, one cell. This is your personal beginning. Depending on the level of stress brought in via the genetic and karmic influences, conception can be quite disturbing.

Each person has their own 'blend' of genetic and karmic influences that enter at conception, which will determine their afferent or efferent orientation. The degree of stress brought in at conception cause some to pull away from life, creating an afferent orientation. Others push forward into life creating an efferent orientation.

The stresses introduced at conception will affect how you develop on all levels in the womb. These stresses create your attitude of mind toward coming into life. Your afferent or efferent orientation will affect how your birthing process goes as well as how you will perceive life from birth onward, including how you will respond or react to the people and situations presented throughout life.

Conception is registered in the first cervical vertebra and directly influences all seven cervical vertebrae. Physically, conception affects the jaw, mouth, throat and neck.

Conception also has an influence on all aspects of a person. The first cell is imprinted at conception. This cell reproduces and influences the rest of the cells that create each individual.

The reflex point is the joint of the big toe and influences down to where the big toe meets the body of the foot.

Post-conception: the 6th - 23rd week of gestation

This period is about growth and development.

All the elements needed to create a new person are present. The task at hand is to grow and develop. One can proceed with the development or procrastinate. The attitude of procrastination can be a pattern throughout life. If the procrastination is extreme, the child is born retarded, meaning held back in development.

Miscarriages tend to take place during this time. Some opt out in this phase, if the idea of coming into life feels too daunting.

Physically, post-conception affects the shoulders, arms, thoracic spine and everything housed from within the top of the shoulders to the diaphragm or base of the rib cage.

The reflex points begin where the big toe meets the ball of the foot to just in front of the inside round ankle bone.

Pre-birth: the 23rd week - birth

This period is about preparing for birth, action and change.

If there is significant underlying stress present during pre-birth the baby may experience feelings of anxiety, frustration or inadequacy. There may be a fear of change, or a resistance to moving forward into the next phase, birth.

These attitudes present during gestation continue to influence you throughout life, operating at an unconscious level. Robert used to say that the prenatal period is a test run for life; how we deal with internal and external stress in the womb is similar to how we will deal with stress throughout life.

Physically, pre-birth influences the area from the diaphragm to the bottom of the pelvis. This encompasses the digestive, elimination and reproductive systems as well as the lumbar spine, sacrum and hips.

The reflex area is from just below the inside ankle bone to just before the edge of the heel.

Birth

Birth relates to the principle of action. This is reflected in your ability or inability to freely move forward in life.

With Metamorphosis we look at the attitudes and nature of any situation. A difficult labor and delivery is often representative of a resistance to coming forward into life or the inability to move into action.

Babies that arrive past their due date, may be reluctant to come forth, or are lacking in the initiative to take action. Premature babies may arrive early because they are ready and excited about coming forward into life. Or, they may arrive early simply because they were anxious to leave the energy of the womb environment.

Physically birth affects the urethra, genital area and coccyx. The reflex point is just before the edge of the heel bone.

The Creation Theme

The creation theme introduces the principles of awareness, concept, idea, thought, form, creation and action. These principles represent the natural movement of awareness into action (or afference into efference.) This is creation, the movement of the essence of life into physical manifestation.

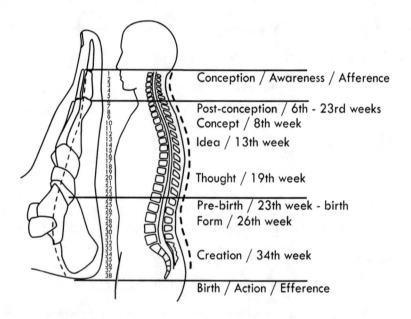

Robert initially diagrammed this with a triangle and later realized that the triangle was part of a sphere. I chose to diagram the theme of the prenatal pattern with the theme of creation to show you how they correspond to the weeks of gestation. Visually, it is helpful to see how it pertains to the actual practice of Metamorphosis.

The purpose of any structure in Metamorphosis is to offer a means to present a theme. It is helpful to have an awareness of this theme and not to consider it as a separate structure. The prenatal pattern and the theme of creation correspond with the weeks of gestation, and together they encompass a greater theme.

The prenatal pattern gives you the theme of development during the phases of gestation and the creation theme offers a means to visualize how awareness moves into action. They both address the attitudes of mind that create our lives.

Awareness is at the same point as conception. This is the first human manifestation of the principle of afference.

Concept is the level of the 8th week. This is the end of the embryonic period; the creation of the primary structure of the body is complete. There is an abstract view of the patterns of life.

Idea is the level of the 13th week. An image formed in the mind which has the potential for structure.

Thought is the level of the 19th week, the 9th thoracic vertebra, the level of the solar plexus. This is where afference and efference blend and cross over. Thought exists but is not prepared for manifestation.

Form is the level of the 26th week. This is the beginning of the potential of physical action. Robert used to equate it with the framework of a house.

Creation is the level of the 34th week, the top of the sacrum. This is when all that is needed for the full manifestation of awareness into action is present; you are preparing for action. This is reflected in your desire and ability to create. Tension in this area is often expressed via sport or sex.

Action is at the same point as birth. This is the principle of action, the ability to move forward in life.

The Afferent-Efferent Dynamic in the Personality

Although it is not necessary to break down the principle of afference and efference, it is helpful to show you how their dynamic occurs in every aspect of life.

Unblocked afference is pure consciousness and awareness. Unblocked efference is action and response. Afference has a thought and efference responds, bringing thought into action or manifestation; they function together. Functioning from unblocked afference and efference is living in the present moment in a state of response to life.

While observing the characteristics of afference and efference in people, there is often a tendency to try to label them. Keep in mind that when you label someone, you no longer truly relate to that person. While everyone has an afferent or efferent orientation, labeling someone as afferent or efferent is not of any benefit. Just as with symptoms and conditions, it is best not to identify with an orientation as it tends to hold you in that pattern.

It is more useful to understand the dynamic between afference and efference and how they manifest in yourself, others and the global environment. The aim of Metamorphosis is to create a balance of afference and efference within. As the two come closer into balance, their relationship becomes more positive, healthy and creative. Put another way, as the tension between the two reduces or ceases to exist, we begin to function more optimally in every way.

Afference or Efference as Your Primary Orientation

At conception, based on your genetic and karmic influences, you take on an afferent or efferent perspective or orientation toward life. This orientation determines how you view life as well as how you interpret and handle the stresses of life. We call it an orientation rather than a tendency because your primary perspective orients you toward how you approach life.

It is important to note that while you have an afferent or efferent orientation, you will experience both afferent and efferent blocks. You also experience afferent and efferent viewpoints throughout the day. You have the ability to 'be' afferent or efferent in any given moment, due to the situations or people present at the time.

Afference and efference are not linear. They function as a dynamic that is operating in every moment and interaction. This explains why we can have an afferent orientation and think or behave efferently, and vice versa.

It is helpful to notice the direction of movement of afference and efference when considering the nature of a block or pattern. In general, due to stress, afference compulsively retreats inward and efference compulsively pushes outward. Keep in mind that stress most often comes from within, due to our underlying stress patterns. We react to external stress based on the level and nature of our internal stress. This stress operates at an unconscious level. We are often unaware that it motivates our choices and affects our well-being as well as our relationships with other people.

The afferently-oriented tend to turn their attention and stress inward, blaming themselves for conflict and painfully recognizing their own flaws. They have a tendency to live life internally, thinking and observing rather than participating. Time spent alone is often preferred to time spent with others. They are inclined to seek guidance and direction from within. Notice that the direction is toward the self or within the self.

The efferently-oriented tend to direct their attention and stress outward, toward others, blaming others for conflict and recognizing everyone else's flaws. They tend to live life in an outward manner, engaging in group activities with less attention on introspection. They are also inclined to seek guidance and direction from outside of the self, often creating a structure of hierarchy when doing so. Notice that the direction is away from the self.

Again, afference and efference are not linear, but you can get an idea of the degree of blockage from the following diagram.

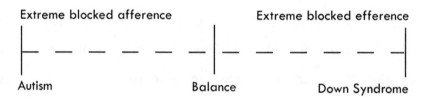

As you get further from the balance of afference and efference your patterns, reactions and degree of internal tension are more extreme. As you get closer to a balance of afference and efference, your patterns, reactions and the degree of internal tension are less extreme. The degree of tension between afference and efference lessens as you come closer to balance. The more in balance you are, the easier it is to experience both afferent and efferent characteristics, positive and negative. The less 'in balance' you are, the more difficult it is to access qualities of the opposite orientation.

When in balance you are able to access the positive qualities of afference and efference as needed, without effort. This is awareness moving into action without hindrance. This is the aim of Metamorphosis, to be able to respond to life as needed in any given moment.

Let me share a story of when this dynamic became clear to me. In 1996 I arranged for Robert to lecture in California. He stayed in our home a week before the lecture, which gave us time to sit and chat about Metamorphosis. Robert, being afferent in nature, communicated in an abstract manner. This required me to absorb the essence of what he was saying rather than to hear information. In order for me to communicate in this manner and tune-in to the nature of Metamorphosis, I went further into afference than I was used to. This was a place where I found great insight into the work.

While I found it very enjoyable to engage with Metamorphosis in this way, the phone frequently rang with requests for me to take care of lecture related details. This required action/efference at a moment's notice. I found it difficult to act upon things and began to feel stressed and tired. Had I been in better balance, I would have been able to naturally respond with what was needed at any given moment, without any stress or effort.

I had many conversations with Robert both that week and on the phone throughout the year prior to the lecture. What was curious about every conversation is that I always walked away thinking, "I wonder what we just talked about?" I could not repeat much of the conversation because it occurred on a different plane. This is how I know that Metamorphosis is absorbed rather than learned.

The Afferent Orientation

Those who are afferently-oriented identify with the principle of life rather than the action of life. It is common to find the afferently-oriented sitting on the sidelines, observing. By standing on the perimeter they avoid interacting with life. This might be seen as someone who avoids engaging in sports, activities and sometimes even conversation. Sometimes the afferently-oriented are so quiet and withdrawn that people do not notice them.

A funny example of how afference is not seen, or in this case heard, is my previous experience with restaurants. When I ate in a restaurant my meal would rarely arrive as ordered. This happened all the time and usually with just my order. I realized that due to my retreative nature my order was just not heard. Thankfully, over time, as I came into better balance, my orders began to arrive as requested.

The extreme expression of the afferent orientation is autism. Consider the nature of those considered to be autistic; they are in a chronic state of retreat. They are extremely sensitive and any external stimulation can be quite overwhelming. They do not like direct eye contact and touch can be very uncomfortable for them. When very stressed they may rock back and forth. They often walk on their tiptoes, as they are not very grounded in life.

The afferently-oriented have a tendency to retreat from life. The retreat can be obvious, such as running away from or avoiding confrontation, stressful people and situations. Or the retreat can be within, sometimes to the extent that they do not hear or notice the people or environment around them. When in retreat it is difficult to communicate. Often the words are in their head but they are unable to get them 'out,' creating frustration for all concerned.

It is not uncommon for an afferently-oriented person to feel attacked by efference, even if it is not an intended attack. To the afferently-oriented person, the energy of efference comes on very strong, as if it is attacking, while the efferent party often thinks they are behaving just fine. The afferently-oriented person will put up with these real or perceived naggings, slights and insults for a while. They will put up with it, overlook it, put up with it and overlook it, until suddenly—due to the build up of tension—they flip into efference and lash out. Their behavior, being uncharacteristic and often extreme to the actual situation, because the tension had built-up, is often perceived by others as over-reactive, irrational or hysterical. The built-up tension is gone, but the frustration of not being heard or understood is often still there. Of course, they will blame themselves for their outburst.

Those who are afferently-oriented tend to be objective in their approach to life and can see many different points of view. When very afferently-oriented, they often cannot have a viewpoint of their own. They have a tendency to be 'wishy-washy.' A more balanced person can see many possibilities or points of view, yet still have one they prefer, while not making it right or needing others to agree.

Afferently-Oriented Children

Because most societal and educational systems are efferent in nature, it is helpful for parents of afferently-oriented children to understand the afferent nature.

The structure of most educational systems is focused on memorizing and reiterating data. Those who are afferently-oriented understand the nature or principle of ideas and are often overwhelmed by data. They see the 'big picture' and do not have the same desire or ability to remember data.

Afferently-oriented children often prefer solo activities and the parents often worry that their children should have more social interaction. Parents frequently push these children into team sports or group activities in an effort to help them.

Forcing afferent children into situations they cannot cope with, even with their best interest at heart, can do more harm than good. Some children are not capable of assuming enough efference and constantly struggle with their perceived 'inadequacies.' Afferently-oriented children, and adults, are very aware of their shortcomings, because their orientation is to look inward. Forcing them into efferent environments may cause them to retreat further.

This is not to suggest that afferent children, or adults, do not desire social activities, but the stress involved may be overwhelming for them.

Receiving Metamorphosis treatments, if the child is open to them, will help bring him into better balance. As a result, the child may naturally seek social activities on his or her own. Children often grasp Metamorphosis right away, so it is possible to teach a child to work on himself, including using the hand symbols. This may be best if the child is old enough to understand what he is doing and/or the parent feels the need for the child to change in some way. If the child is feeling external pressure to change, he will most likely retreat even further. Finding a practitioner or teaching the child to work on himself removes the pressure from all concerned.

Sometimes it is obvious that something is bothering an afferent child and a more efferent parent may ask what is wrong. If the child is very afferent, he will retreat from the efference of the question. We have all seen a movie or television program where a father takes his son fishing and just sits with him. The boy, finally able to relax, begins to share what is on his mind. The efferent presence and pressure is gone.

It is helpful for parents to understand the nature of afference and efference and know that afferently-oriented children and adults can be quite happy, even if they are not conforming to the norm. It is usually better to encourage people to be who they are, without focusing on negative perceptions of what they 'are not' or how they 'should' be. If this is a struggle for the parents, Metamorphosis treatments may be helpful for them too.

Afference in the Movies

Bruce Lee brought the perspective of no technique, or tuning-in, to the martial arts. The movie *A Warrior's Journey* is a documentary-style movie that portrays his philosophy. The concept of the movie is that Bruce fights his way up the floors of a pagoda. On each floor he is met by an opponent, each one trained in a different style of martial arts. He bests each opponent because he tunes-in to every situation and functions with awareness, rather than a trained style. While his philosophy is not the same as Robert's, they both embody tuning-in or working with awareness rather than technique. I found it fascinating to watch this concept displayed in physical form.

Dustin Hoffman portrayed the extreme disturbance of afference in the movie *Rain Man*. The character was very intelligent, yet he could not function in the day-to-day aspects of life and required constant care.

Russell Crowe portrayed the extreme discomfort the afferently-oriented can feel in social situations in the movie *A Beautiful Mind*. The character he portrayed was an extremely intelligent man who suffered from schizo-phrenia, an extreme afferent pattern.

A Summary of Afferent Characteristics

- Creative
- Relates to the principle of life
- Independence of mind, thinks for oneself
- Objective, able to see many points of view
- Intuitive, inner knowing
- Uses structure only as needed
- Non-linear thinkers
- Tendency to be disorganized
- Retreats within under stress, internalizes
- Victim pattern, covertly and overtly attacked due to their retreative nature
- Blames oneself rather than others
- Tends to tiptoe around, preferring not to draw attention to oneself
- Feels unheard and has a hard time speaking up
- Often feels like they don't belong or fit in
- Prefers quiet activities alone or with small groups
- Mental tension and illness are afferent in nature

The Efferent Orientation

While the afferently-oriented relate to the principle of life, the efferently-oriented relate to the action of life. They like to be 'actively' involved with life, often engaging in a busy social life, playing team sports, belonging to clubs and participating in group activities. They tend to be drawn to structured organizations and are often attracted to leadership positions. They are comfortable with, and often seek, the spotlight.

Efferently-oriented people encourage conformity and tend to resent the independence of mind, or non-conforming nature, of the afferently-oriented. Conformity is a large part of all efferently structured organizations, such as government, business, education and religion.

The extreme expression of the efferent orientation is Down Syndrome. Those considered to be Down Syndrome are easily recognizable, as this pattern causes the facial features to appear somewhat pushed 'outward.' Robert used the word retarded in reference to this pattern, which is used in its literal sense to mean held back in their development. This is due to the attitude of procrastination, which would have begun at or around conception. Often their level of development, even as an adult, remains that of an adolescent or child. They tend to be outgoing and enjoy people.

A more efferently-oriented person, under stress, will often lash out at others, verbally or physically. Someone else would be at fault, of course, for the efferently-oriented project the blame outward. The lashing outward is compulsive, an immediate reaction to the situation, that is soon forgotten. (While the afferent party, subject to their attack, is often stunned into retreat.)

The efferently-oriented tend to lack objectivity and can only see one point of view on any topic. Their point of view is the 'right' one, which is the 'truth!' This is the attitude of mind that is behind much of the conflict in the world.

People fight for what they believe is a religious, moral or political truth that they strongly believe in. This creates tension, chaos, judgment and war.

People also argue and alienate others due to their beliefs. Gay marriage is a hot topic at the moment. While people argue over the belief that they feel is 'right' they lose perspective about what is important. Love, commitment and the needs of the individuals get lost in the argument.

This tension is also seen in the healing arts, creating a division of practitioners with differing beliefs. The negative relationship between afference and efference keeps people disconnected, alienated and arguing.

The efferently-oriented tend to view things in terms of right or wrong and true or false. They also feel compelled to back their beliefs with data and proof. However, research is typically biased in one way or another and a researcher can use 'facts' to his advantage.

I once attended a lecture discussing cellular intelligence. The speaker ended his presentation with the statement, "...we must continue to collect the data to prove that which we already know." I found this to be a humorous example of the efferent perspective.

The Efferently-Oriented Child

Efferently-oriented children are fortunate that the structure of education, religion and social norms are created by the efferently-oriented. Most educational systems are structured on the concept of memorizing and reiterating data rather than considering the nature of, or principles behind, ideas. The system of giving grades, participating in team sports and encouraging competition are efferent concepts. The efferently-oriented child is likely to appreciate, understand and enjoy these activities.

A more efferent child will feel the urge to verbally or physically attack a more afferent child. The child that bullies and the child that is bullied are both subject to the compulsive dynamic of negative afference and efference.

Efference in the Movies

The concept of a movie is efferent, as it is the image of, or the imitation of, life.

Some movies are based on character development and depict the afferent-efferent dynamic that cause our personal and global dilemmas. Those who are efferently-oriented love movies with lots of violence, sex and special effects, designed to stimulate a person rather than portray a story.

The most obvious efferent characters are in 'action' movies such as *Rambo* or *The Terminator*.

A Summary of Efferent Characteristics

- Finds ease in communication
- Relates to the existing structure of life
- Is comfortable with the activities of daily life
- Organized, linear thinkers
- Data-oriented, needs scientific or documented proof, fond of facts
- Enjoys group, team or social activities, often in leadership roles
- Group-minded and conforming, often resents independent thinking
- Uses structure for the sake of structure, often creating hierarchy in the process
- Lacks creativity, copies rather than originates
- Lacks objectivity, unable to see more than one point of view

- Often draws attention to oneself through ones actions and tendency to speak loudly
- Prefers loud or busy activities with lots of people
- Perpetrator pattern
- Projects blame outward toward others
- When upset, lashes outward toward others, verbally or physically
- Physical, behavioral and emotional disturbances are efferent in nature

Different Variations of Efference

• Forced Efference

Forced efference is a temporary forcing of efference for a period of time, such as to give a lecture or attend a party. This can occur consciously or unconsciously. The person manages to get through the event or situation, but with incredible effort. This forcing of efference is not natural and expends a lot of energy.

• Conditioned Efference

Conditioned efference occurs when an afferently-oriented person learns to assume efference as their primary mode of function. Because most educational and societal structures are efferent, children are often pushed into an efferent mode of function at an early age. This mode of function tends to unconsciously continue through life as they get used to this conditioned orientation. The efferent orientation fits well into the hierarchy and structure of the business world, the corporate ladder, company rules and required ways of doing things.

The price to pay for conditioned efference is often illness, because people are regularly forcing more energy than they actually have. Most likely they are very tired at the end of the day or possibly depend on caffeine or other stimulants. Efference is action, so the efferently-oriented or those in good balance have much more energy for 'doing' things than the afferently-oriented, which tend to think about doing things.

It can be very liberating for someone who is conditioned with efference to recognize this acquired mode of function. Afferently-oriented people do not 'follow the grain' well; they like to do things a little differently and do not appreciate the viewpoints of hierarchy or unnecessary structure.

• Sub Efference

Sub efference is the absence of afference, consciousness and light. Often this is expressed in hard core drug addiction, serial killings or participation in devil worship. It is hard, but not impossible, for people who have gone this far away from afference (consciousness) to find their way out. This pattern is often portrayed in horror movies or movies considered to have a dark element to them.

• Rogue Efference

Rogue efference pertains to those with a compulsive need for frequent sexual activity. Due to their unconscious, underlying tension they usually need something extra or unusual to push past the tension and reach climax. This pattern, in all its variations and themes, is often portrayed in pornographic magazines and movies.

The Afferent-Efferent Dynamic
in Relationships

Robert said that relationships were primarily based on the affinity of chaos, meaning that people are drawn together by their blocks and negative patterns. Initially, the negative patterns seem to disappear, creating the sense of falling in love. This is often experienced as euphoria, that overwhelming feeling of joy and aliveness. As time goes on, the temporary balance disappears and their patterns come into full play. This is commonly noted as the end of the honeymoon! Couples begin to fight about little things because they are struggling with the underlying tensions within themselves and the dynamic of negative afference and efference.

Borrowed Afference & Efference

People unconsciously borrow from the ability of the opposite orientation from another person, most often their partner. The more afferent person relies on the efference of another to get things done or to accompany them to social functions. Socially the afferently-oriented tend to cling as they need to borrow efference in order to be there. This is what some term the co-dependent pattern, when you need the orientation of another person in order to fully function.

The more efferent person tends to rely on the creativity and awareness of another, often looking to a more afferent person for insight, ideas or answers to their problems.

When we partner, this borrowing takes place all the time and resentment begins to build. Often we do not know why our partners are so annoying to us, because this dynamic is occurring unconsciously.

This dynamic can also occur in any relationship, with a friend, co-worker or family member. This is a common dynamic with business partners. The afferently-oriented person comes up with an idea but they do not have enough efference to do much with it. The tendency is to partner with a more efferently-oriented person who will finance and/or bring their idea out into the world. This explains how many healing arts have become so efferent in nature. The efferent partner, in an attempt to market the idea, often loses the afference or essence of the work.

Assumed Afference & Efference

Everyone has an orientation, which is evident by how you typically deal with stress. You also experience both afferent and efferent perspectives. If an afferent person is with someone who is more afferent than they are, they temporarily assume efference in relation to that person or situation. If an efferent person is with a person more efferent than they are, they temporarily assume afference in relation to that person or situation. This dynamic fluctuates within a partnership and in all interactions. Remember afference and efference are not linear. They function together at all times in relation to each other. You constantly and unconsciously participate in this dynamic based on your orientation, what you are doing and who you are with.

Observing this dynamic within yourself creates an opportunity to really understand the nature of each orientation. It also helps you see the bigger picture, as you begin to see the compulsive nature of afference and efference and all the dysfunction their negative relationship creates.

The Relationship Pattern

The nature of the function of the genitalia has an effect on male-female relationships. This pattern seems to become more deeply ingrained over time. Robert's theory on the relationship pattern is based on the function of the genitalia for reproduction. Men initiate pregnancy with ejaculation. The female body responds and then completes the act by carrying and delivering a child.

Afference initiates and efference responds; this is their dynamic. As afference initiates, the male is subject to the afferent pattern in relation to his female partner. As efference responds, the female is subject to the efferent pattern in relationship to her male partner. A woman can be afferently-oriented, but unconsciously assumes efference in relationship to her partner and vice versa. This dynamic is present, but is less extreme, when the partners are of the same sex.

A typical scenario in marriage is the husband who comes home, sits in his chair and does not communicate much. His wife, either curious how his day went or in reaction to his retreat, begins to ask questions. Questions are efferent in nature, so he starts to feel attacked or interrogated and retreats further within, finding it harder and harder to communicate. She, on the other hand, is pushed further into efference and pursues her line of questioning, often more aggressively. Thus, the cycle of nagging begins, with complaints such as "you never talk to me..." As efference tends to be very repetitive, she will begin to say this over and over, day after day.

It is helpful if each partner realizes that both patterns are compulsive and unpleasant. It is stressful to be in retreat, unable to communicate or function as desired. It is equally as stressful to be in reaction to the retreat.

No one likes to be the nagger or attacker any more than they like to be nagged or attacked. To be compelled into efference is stressful and takes its toll on that person, especially if they have an afferent orientation.

Because these patterns are compulsive, your partner's actions are not necessarily an expression of how he or she feels about you. Understanding this will spare both parties a lot of frustration and hurt feelings.

The obvious solution to this relationship pattern would be to practice Metamorphosis on yourself and/or each other. As each person can better access both afference and efference within, they cease to borrow from each other, thus reducing unconscious resentment.

If you are in an unhappy relationship, working on yourself will either create less tension between you and your partner, or one of you will find it easier to leave. The efferent partner is usually the one that leaves or moves 'out.'

Ideally, if both parties come into reasonable balance, the relationship will be based on friendship and appreciation of one another, rather than 'an affinity of chaos.'

The Sex/Sensuality Pattern

The sex pattern is compulsive and exists within everyone to some degree. There is often a lot of shame, guilt and judgment around this particular pattern.

The sex pattern is indeed one of humanity's primary stress patterns. All we have to do is look at advertising to see how easy it is to sell almost anything if you appeal to the sex drive. We actually call it a drive, for some are driven to find release from the tension. The fact that there is tension indicates there is stress involved.

The primary function of the reproductive organs is to reproduce, yet most often sex is based on the need to relieve tension and/or to experience pleasure. The sensuality pattern introduced pleasure to the sexual act beyond its primary function. For some, the need for this pleasure is compulsive and they frequently seek sexual gratification. This is popularly known as sex addiction. Others try to over-ride their compulsions by attempting celibacy.

Those functioning from a block at the thirty-fourth week, at the hip level, often require extra stimulation in order to push through this block and reach climax. We can all think of a few things that people use or do to increase excitement. For some, this pattern is extreme and may lead them to pursue what is considered as unacceptable sexual behavior, often involving pain, degradation, or sex with unwilling or inappropriate partners such as children or animals. What is helpful to remember is that although the person engaging in these acts does experience pleasure, they are also suffering from tremendous tension.

Physically, tension from the coccyx will radiate out and affect the male genitalia. The coccyx represents action, thus men often experience a frequent need for sexual activity. The more efferently-oriented often channel this energy into sports or engage in promiscuous activity. The more afferently-oriented often engage in self-pleasuring with the help of pornography. The internet or phone sex is a perfect medium for this pattern. Keep in mind the nature of patterns; the afferent pattern is often uncomfortable being with people yet they are still subject to sexual tension

The female genitalia and the womb, in relation to the spine, sit closer to the sacrum. This gives women a different perspective on sex. Females frequently experience this tension as their 'biological clock' and/or menstrual problems. For many women, their biological clock ticks away and they feel the need to become mothers, even though they may not be ready for or truly interested in that lifestyle. Menstruation is a natural function of the body yet most women experience symptoms of emotional and physical stress at some point in their cycles.

This pattern affects women sexually as well. Women often find pleasure in being, or feel compelled to be, the object of desire. Sex could not be an industry if we did not have women who are the sexy or pornographic models and actresses, exotic dancers, prostitutes and sexual enticers. Keep in mind that this is also a stress pattern.

Sex is a lucrative industry that caters to this pattern. Sex can be found in books, magazines, the movies, television and via the internet and telephone. Jails are full of perpetrators, those who suffer with the efferent aspect of the pattern. Many children and adults live with the emotional pain caused by the afferent aspect of the pattern, being the victim. Public and religious figures are often under scrutiny for this pattern. It would be wonderful if people recognized that punishing this pattern does not resolve it. The pattern needs to be addressed for what it is, an imbalance of afference and efference. Then we will not have to find ways to protect our victims and punish our perpetrators, for there won't be any!

For those of you that are getting worried, this is not to suggest that sexual activity will cease to exist, just the negative and compulsive aspects of the pattern. This leaves more room for genuine intimacy.

The Afferent-Efferent Dynamic and Abuse

The afferent pattern is the victim and the efferent pattern is the perpetrator.

Afference retreats from the energy of efference. The act of moving away from efference elicits efference to move outward in a negative manner. Afference initiates and efference responds. In the negative pattern, afference retreats and is often victimized and efference reacts and is often the perpetrator.

All of this occurs on an unconscious level, so neither party is entirely aware of the dynamic that takes place. Victims of attack often feel they are to blame. Because of their inner, afferent awareness, they realize they played a role in the dynamic.

Of course, this is not the same thing as suggesting that the person deserved the attack or that it was their fault. This is the result of the negative relationship between afference and efference. Both patterns are compulsive and both parties are blocked and suffering.

Child abuse is often directed toward one child in a family. This child is usually the most afferent, eliciting the attack from the most efferent member of the family. Remember that people assume an orientation in relation to one another. For example, a man who is afferent in relation to his wife can be efferent in relation to a child who is more afferent than he is.

The Image Pattern

The image pattern is humanity's pattern of looking outside of the self for salvation, guidance and healing.

My intent here is to give you the overall essence of this theme so that you understand the thinking behind the principles and practice.

Robert goes into greater detail in his collection of *Introductory Articles*.

Robert observed that time, space, our universe and humanity were created from the separation of afference and efference; from oneness into duality. He was not sure if this separation occurred by accident or by choice, as a means to work through a flaw in the overall pattern.

Due to the separation, efference turned away from afference and expanded outward. This created time, the universe and life as we know it.

> 66
> . . . Afferent and Efferent. These two names provide us with a "channel" of thought from the beginning of the cause of the stress— sometimes from the beginning of time. To analyze this in detail was only necessary in the first place to be able to create the symbol.
> —Robert St. John
> 99

The creation of time allows for stress to be carried through time, via genetic and karmic patterns. Karmic patterns reside in time and space and have affected humanity from the beginning of time. Genetic patterns are passed on via our maternal and paternal genes and have also affected humanity from the beginning of time.

The separation of afference and efference created a disturbance in their relationship and is the initial and primary stress pattern of humanity. All disturbances we individually and collectively experience are due to the tension between afference and efference.

The image pattern is a result of this separation. As efference turned away it began expanding outward. As a result, afference (consciousness) went into abeyance or retreat. With afference in abeyance, efference began to create consciousness from the image of, or memory of, afference. Due to the nature of efference, it created the image of afference outside of itself. This became the basis for religion, to look to a superior being outside and above the self for salvation and guidance. It also became the basis for the hierarchical structure of looking to experts outside and above the self for healing.

Just a note: Robert often used analogy as a means to impart a theme. I tend to consider the separation of afference and efference to be an analogy rather than an actual event. Meaning, the theme isn't meant to become a creation story. I think the insight of the relationship between afference and efference is what is important.

It is helpful to remember that Metamorphosis is about looking at the greater theme of life and bringing that awareness into your perspective, so that it translates into your practice. There is always a bit of 'mystery' in life that does not need to be nailed down. The theme is to create an awareness within you, which opens the door, so to speak, to creating a balance of afference and efference within yourself.

The Image Pattern in Spirituality and Religion

We are naturally connected to the consciousness of life and our inner intelligence at all times, but do not always feel, remember, or know that. Due to our blocks, we experience a separation from consciousness and thus often seek it outside of ourselves.

Consider the nature of religion and spirituality in relationship to looking outside the self for guidance or salvation. Religions worship a god, several gods, or a revered figure. There is usually dogma or discipline involved, often requiring a denial of pleasure or a repression of 'negative' patterns.

The New Age movement is often part of the image pattern. People look to the Great Spirit, the Universe, the Goddess, other deities, beings or dimensions. Gurus, masters and people who channel for other beings and universes are often sought out.

This is not to suggest that any of the above do not exist, have value or purpose. The theme here is to consider how we view ourselves to be separate from consciousness.

We are naturally connected to the source of greater consciousness. Our blocks create a sense of separation but we are not separate. The idea with Metamorphosis is that as you come closer to a balance of afference and efference, your blocks clear and you recognize that you are connected to higher consciousness. This is when your life really starts to change.

People often ask if they need to give up their spiritual or religious beliefs to practice Metamorphosis. Metamorphosis is about thinking for yourself and encourages independence of mind over dogma and conditioned thinking. It is always a good idea to look at the nature of the thinking behind what you believe and what you are considering working with, so that your choices are made with greater awareness. Take the time to really look at the perspectives, modalities and philosophies in your life to see if they are truly in alignment with how you want to approach your life.

Robert used to say that people 'give things up' when they were ready to. This includes Metamorphosis practitioners, because you can work on yourself.

I tend to see this theme as finding a balance between respecting greater consciousness and personal responsibility. To me, this is the balance of afference and efference. This balance is what is needed for global transformation. When all forms of life recognize and experience this consciousness our planet will transform itself.

I practice Metamorphosis as my primary approach to increasing consciousness. I appreciate the emphasis on personal responsibility as well as the simplicity of the practice. I view Metamorphosis as trusting the innate intelligence to align itself with greater consciousness, and in doing so, create better health and a more fulfilling life.

Keep in mind that we are in an exciting time right now, where there are more options then ever to assist us with connecting to our inner guidance. Metamorphosis is a nice, simple way to do this. Metamorphosis is not meant to become or replace a belief system. It is about freeing yourself from conditioned thinking and living fully in the present.

> **"**
>
> Although Metamorphosis is an attitude of mind and very
> simple to use, we have been indoctrinated over the centuries
> by structures of thought in religion, philosophy and education
> in such a way that our ability to think and function from the level
> of thought is tied to these same structures and we are not free
> to 'think' from our own inner intelligence. We need some ritual to
> 'unthink' this structure. That, in principle, is what Metamorphosis is.
> What physical practice there is in Metamorphosis is a symbol
> for the mind to change all of the indoctrination of the
> past and to 'become' the present.
>
> **"**
>
> —An excerpt from the article, *The Metamorphosis Centre*
> by Robert St. John

The Image Pattern and the Nature of Healing

Since the beginning of time, humanity has been looking to an outside source for healing, whether the approach has been conventional or alternative.

This section invites you to consider the nature of healing in general, so that when you make choices regarding your health and well-being, it is done with greater awareness.

The perspective of Metamorphosis is that your inner intelligence has the ability to heal from within. Healing is a natural response to creating a balance of afference and efference, rather than the aim. This idea is important to understand the intent of Metamorphosis.

To understand how intention is used in the healing arts it is helpful to observe the thinking behind different approaches. Begin to look at the scope of the intention of different modalities. Reflexologists have often asked why they do not experience change in all areas of their life as they also work on the spinal reflex points. Although Reflexology is not of the image pattern, because it recognizes that the body is self-healing, it is limited by its scope of intention. When reflex points are used with the intent to heal on a physical level, you will experience change at the physical level.

People often try to mix Reflexology and Metamorphosis together. This does not work because the intentions are very different, which is apparent by how different their charts are.

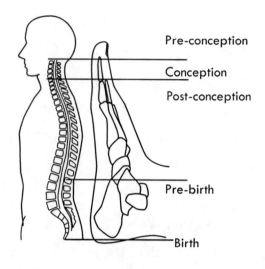

Prenatal Pattern ©

Metamorphosis and Reflexology only share the concept of reflex points. Metamorphosis uses the spinal reflex points as symbols for the prenatal pattern and theme of Metamorphosis. This enables you to create a balance of afference and efference within. The intent of Metamorphosis is to let go of the underlying patterns that create our individual and global disturbances. Although both approaches use the ancient concept of reflex points, they have different maps and intentions and thus different outcomes.

Reflexology, as well as quite a few other approaches, recognizes that the body is self-healing. With Metamorphosis we recognize that the innate intelligence is capable of changing our attitudes of mind. This creates a more positive approach to life and thus we cease to create illness, suffering and conflict. Rather than working with the body we are working with the underlying attitudes that create dysfunction, disharmony and disease. Although this may seem like a bantering of words, it is the fine-tuning of your intent that determines the nature of the outcome.

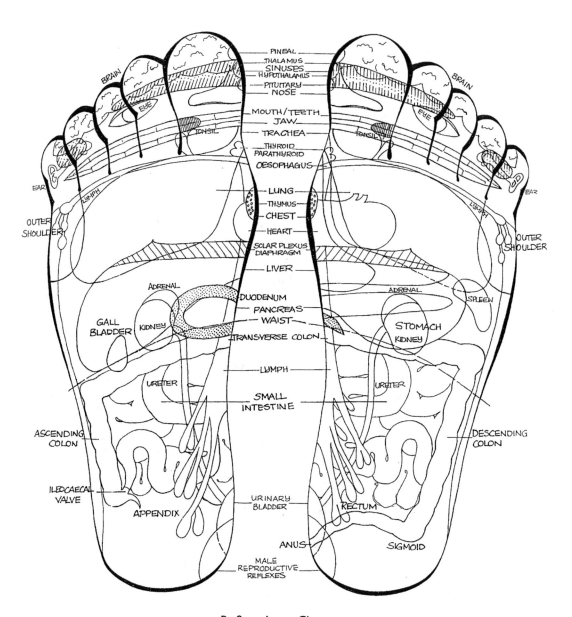

Reflexology Chart
West Australian School of Reflexology ©

Consider the different scopes of intention in regard to treating symptoms. By treating mental, emotional, behavioral, spiritual or physical symptoms, we create an array of approaches, all limited in their scope of intention. The more complicated healing becomes the less effective it usually is.

Consider the scope of intention in relation to time. Does the approach look back to childhood, birth, conception, or a past life? The scope of the intention for Metamorphosis goes back to the creation of time, space and humanity's primary stress patterns. These patterns are carried through time via the genetic and karmic patterns. From this perspective, to address a moment in time is symptomatic.

Most therapies aim to re-condition the mind with dialogue, affirmations and regression work, which often rely on the intellect and skill of the therapist. Metamorphosis un-conditions the mind rather than re-conditions it, letting go of our limiting patterns so that we may function optimally on all levels. The thinking here is that as the underlying pattern goes the stress and trauma associated with the pattern also leaves. By un-conditioning the mind we truly begin to think for ourselves, with more independence of mind.

People frequently ask if they need to give up receiving other modalities while receiving Metamorphosis. The idea is to increase your level of awareness, not give-up something that you find helpful or useful in your life.

Robert said that, in general, receiving one modality at a time is most effective. This gives you the time needed to complete a treatment, as many approaches continue to work after the treatment is over. The other benefit is that you can easily tell what is working. If an approach is not helping, then try a different one.

The healing arts have become very eclectic. Some practitioners mix several modalities together in one treatment and some clients receive several different modalities within a short period of time. Mixing modalities often creates chaos.

As mentioned before, it is always useful to consider the nature of what you are deciding to do. Robert did suggest that you will get the most benefit from Metamorphosis treatments if you do not receive other modalities at the same time. This includes mixing modalities into one treatment as well as receiving other modalities throughout the duration of Metamorphosis treatments. Keep in mind that while this was his observation, he was not in favor of telling people what they should do.

I find it helpful to do what feels right at the time. I have gained an understanding of the nature of healing in general simply by taking notice of the principles and practice behind other modalities and observing how I felt when I received them. Objectively observing increases awareness.

It is helpful to look at your motive when choosing an approach to healing. The motive to use a modality or product to temporarily relieve a symptom is different than using a modality or product to heal at the level of a symptom. Give this some thought!

Healing is really quite simple and may not need to be approached in several ways at once. I encourage you to explore this idea as you may gain a deeper understanding of the nature of healing, motive and intention.

Remember that one of Robert's observations was that humanity's primary patterns of suffering, illness and global disharmony have never really changed. For this reason, using a healing approach that is of the image pattern defeats the intent of Metamorphosis. You can get profound symptomatic change when mixing Metamorphosis with other approaches, but the negative relationship of afference and efference does not change. Thus, collectively we are all still in the same boat.

Keep in mind that Metamorphosis is not a miracle cure-all. In theory, we can change simply by deciding to. Often there is an unconscious resistance to change, due to the tension between afference and efference within yourself. Sometimes our patterns move out very quickly and sometimes they take time.

The Image Pattern in Nutrition, Addiction and Illness

• *Nutrition and Diet*

Food is outside of the self, yet we are dependent on it for survival.

An interesting topic to consider is nutrition or diet. The foods you choose to eat affect your well-being. You can enhance your health by eating well, which is often a task too big for many to accomplish. Many people who have attempted to change their diet for weight loss or health reasons know how challenging it can be to give up the foods they love and crave.

With Metamor-phosis, the idea is that as you come into balance, you naturally desire foods that are healthy and right for your body type. The difference is that there isn't any struggle or effort involved in changing your diet. It is not the goal, for this would be a symptomatic approach, but rather the result. If you stop to think about it, if people were in balance, they would not want to eat unhealthy or unnatural foods. We tend to eat in alignment with our patterns. Have you ever noticed that when you are stressed you eat more junk food? How we choose to eat on a daily basis follows the same principle, but the stress is unconscious, due to our underlying patterns. Thus, we do not realize that this is what motivates our food choices.

• *Addictions*

Addiction is the compulsive need to rely on something outside of the self as a means to cope with our unconscious, internal stress.

People can be addicted to food, chocolate, caffeine, cigarettes, alcohol, drugs, sex, work and more. The nature of addiction is the same regardless of

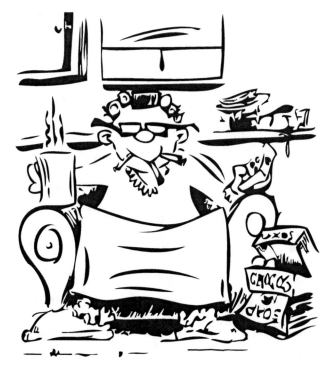

Survival Patterns!

the vice. Often the person is not physically addicted, but rather, is subject to a compulsive pattern as a means of coping. The feeling of need is real, but the need is for a coping mechanism rather than the vice of choice. As we come into balance, we no longer need to rely on things outside of ourselves as a means to cope. The cravings and behavior simply go away without effort.

In general, Robert used to say, "enjoy your sin," meaning, if you are going to engage in an activity, then really enjoy it. Most of us have a vice we wish we could overcome, but we do it anyway, often worrying about it before, during and after. But we still do it! By doing it and letting yourself enjoy it, you take the pressure off yourself. Work on yourself to address the underlying pattern once you are done. (This is the key!)

You can put a lot of effort and determination into trying to give up an addictive pattern, often without long-term success. This is why dieting or forced sobriety is frequently unsuccessful. If you do manage to give up the vice, more often than not you will replace it with another, because the underlying pattern was not addressed.

Metamorphosis is a nice alternative to this struggle. Once the underlying pattern is gone so is the compulsive behavior. I have seen this for myself. When I was fourteen years old I began a challenging pattern of alcohol, drug and cigarette use/abuse which lasted for twelve years, which is when I discovered Metamorphosis. I was a very compulsive, heavy drinker and once I had a drink, I continued until I blacked out, which I did regularly. After receiving Metamorphosis treatments, the compulsive need for all these substances ceased to exist.

Watching that pattern simply leave my life inspired me to learn this work, and is the reason I am so passionate about it. Eighteen years later I am able to enjoy a social drink on occasion without any repercussion and I have never experienced the desire for drugs or cigarettes since. This is contradictory to the common thinking on addiction. It is possible to move out of the pattern and not struggle with it for the rest of your life.

In some instances a physical addiction does occur and depending on the situation, it may be a different picture. This may require effort and detoxification, but Metamorphosis can still help with the overall pattern. Sometimes people may think they are physically addicted because the desire is so strong, but it may simply be the compulsive nature of the imbalance. If this is your pattern, you will have to determine the best avenue to pursue.

• *Physical Illness and Discomfort*

We often seek healing and relief from discomfort outside of the self.

The thinking with Metamorphosis is that the underlying tension in the spine radiates out and disturbs what is in its region. This explains why products and treatments that address physical problems often provide temporary relief.

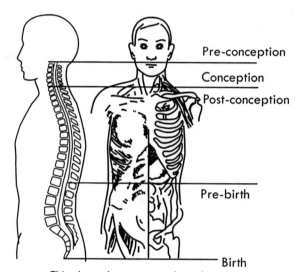

Pre-conception
Conception
Post-conception
Pre-birth
Birth

This chart demonstrates how the
underlying stress in the spine radiates
out and affects the physical body.
This is a re-creation of one of St. John's charts.

Tension in the pre-conception area of the head may create discomfort or illness in relation to the head, brain, ears, eyes, nose and sinuses.

Tension in the conception area of the spine may radiate out and create discomfort or illness in relationship to the jaw, mouth, throat and neck.

Tension in the post-conception area of the spine may radiate out and create discomfort or illness in relationship to the shoulders, upper and mid-back, ribs, arms, chest area, lungs, diaphragm and heart.

Tension in the pre-birth area of the spine may radiate out and create discomfort or illness in relationship to the low back, hips, sacrum, digestive, elimination and reproductive systems. Stress in this area can cause the discomfort related to menstruation.

Tension in the birth area of the spine may radiate out and create discomfort or illness in relationship to the coccyx, legs, knees, ankles and feet.

In relation to the spine, underlying stress causes the cervical, thoracic and lumbar vertebrae, sacrum and coccyx to go out of alignment. Mental tension creates muscular tension, which cause muscles to contract and pull vertebrae out of alignment. Those who suffer from this problem know that the same vertebra keep going out of alignment, because the underlying pattern is not being addressed. The body adjusts itself when there is no underlying tension inhibiting this natural process.

We often experience accidents and injuries to areas with underlying stress. The body is designed to be self-healing. We do not always heal completely when underlying tension is inhibiting this natural process.

• *Afference-Efference and Ill Health*

The Metamorphosis perspective views illnesses and conditions to be caused by the tension between afference and efference. If the illness is mental, it would be considered afferent in nature. If the illness is physical, it would be considered efferent in nature. Of course, it is not necessary to analyze an illness, but it is helpful in gaining an understanding of the nature of negative afference and efference. I have listed a few patterns below so you can begin to see how illness manifests from this perspective.

Anxiety Disorder/Panic Attacks: anxiety is generated and fueled by negative thinking, usually thoughts that you are unaware of. These negative thoughts tend to be about yourself. This constant negative thinking and retreative nervous energy are afferent in nature. A panic attack occurs when the mind interprets these thoughts as a real threat and a physical reaction takes place, flooding the body with adrenaline.

Chronic Fatigue: is a chronic afferent retreat from the action (efference) of life. Just the thought of action, even getting off the sofa or out of bed, can be exhausting.

Bipolar or Manic Depressive Disorder: is an extreme flipping of polarities between afference and efference.

Keep in mind that Metamorphosis does not aim to cure. If you have a serious condition you will need to decide what course of action to take.

Afference-Efference and the Global Dynamic

All life on this planet including animals and the environment, are subject to, or affected by, the tension between afference and efference.

The negative dynamic of afference and efference is behind the nature of all war and disharmony on our planet. Consider how this imbalance affects all living things. Many animals are subjected to domestication, captivity, factory farming, cloning and animal testing. Much of the environment is subject to pollution, strip mining, urbanization, nuclear testing, genetic engineering and global warming—just to name a few problems.

Efference is often well-intended even though the actions may lack awareness. Factory farming can produce a larger quantity of food for a growing population. Animal testing helps find 'cures' for illnesses. If humanity as a whole were in balance, we would not have over-population or illnesses that need cures. We would not have the inclination toward solutions that involve pain and suffering.

Countries, like people, have relationships with each other that are also subject to the negative dynamic of afference and efference. Just as on the personal level, the dynamic of efference attacking afference occurs on the global level. The more efferent countries attack and often overtake countries that are more afferent than they are. Although a geographically small country, England has conquered many different countries and cultures throughout history.

Countries reflect the overall orientation of the land and its inhabitants. Consider the nature of the native animals, as they reflect the orientation of the land. As with people, the afferently-oriented animals tend to be vegetarian and the efferently-oriented animals tend to be carnivores.

The land of Australia is very afferent, with the native Aborigines being an extremely afferent race. Aborigines are an ancient race, yet they have never created permanent structures of any kind. In contrast the Australian culture is affected by the afference of the land and often produces a false 'machismo.'

Look at the nature of the psyche and culture of each country. For example, as countries, England, Holland, Germany and the United States have an efferent orientation. Countries that tend toward capitalism, technology and warfare are efferent in nature.

Consider how much influence Hollywood has on the world. Hollywood is the epitome of the image pattern, as movies are the imitation of life. The United States, via Hollywood, influences much of the world with its culture and viewpoints. The United States also frequently imposes its political views and agendas on other countries.

The Way Out of the Negative Patterns of Afference and Efference

You can spend an endless amount of time and energy helping with worthwhile causes, with so many dilemmas to choose from, but in the big picture, nothing changes. The patterns will find a new outlet and thus new causes, new victims and new saviors. The cycle does not end this way.

> "
> Working on your own patterns is the most effective way to create personal and global peace and harmony.
> "

By working on yourself at a fundamental level, you are effecting change in the overall pattern of negative afference and efference. As more people begin to work at this level, the underlying patterns that create disharmony, suffering and illness will cease to exist.

In 1993 Robert observed that afference and efference returned to their original state. (Please refer to the "Suffix to the Functional Human" at the end of the book for Robert St. John's list of relevant dates.) Efference, which has been dominant since the beginning of human existence is now subject to afference again. As a result, afference as consciousness is shining light onto the negative patterns of humanity, so to speak.

As we enter into the twenty-first century we are moving from the Piscean age into the Aquarian age. With efference in resistance to this, humanity's patterns are currently rising to the surface, causing disasters, chaos, unrest and upheaval.

Metamorphosis is here to assist with this transition. Robert used to say that you are less affected by the chaos around you when you have a good balance of afference and efference. As we individually let go of the patterns of the past, we will collectively move into a more conscious and peaceful existence.

It is helpful to understand the positive and negative nature of afference and efference, their dynamic together, and the patterns they create. Realizing the compulsive nature of patterns allows for more compassion toward yourself and others. As we begin to understand the nature of our own patterns, we will have more unconditional love and compassion for others, for we all have challenging patterns. It is also helpful for parents to understand the afferent-efferent dynamic when making decisions on behalf of their children.

People are often in a hurry to be something 'better' than they are, and do not always appreciate who they already are. Understanding that we are not our patterns reduces the need to be something or someone we are not.

Metamorphosis is ultimately about unconditional love, something we all appreciate receiving but often find hard to give. Judgment is negative efference and the opposite of unconditional love. If we had less judgment for the patterns humanity struggles with, we might be in a better place to let go of them. I find it is helpful to view people with patterns, rather than label them with problems.

In summary, the patterns of abuse, dysfunction, illness and suffering have existed on the planet since the beginning of time. As you address the universal patterns of humanity within yourself, you are also affecting the quality of life on this planet. This means that the best thing you can do to help others, animals, the environment or global disharmony, is to work on yourself.

The Practice

Use your intuition as you work,
let your hands guide you instead of your mind

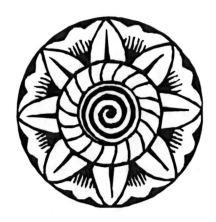

The practice of Metamorphosis is very simple. The principles and theme previously discussed are inherent in your decision to practice Metamorphosis. This allows the practitioner to simply be present with the person receiving the treatment. Metamorphosis is non-verbal and non-directive.

The practice of Metamorphosis includes touching the spinal reflex points on the feet, hands and head as well as working directly on the spine. The hand symbols are also part of the practice. To differentiate, I refer to working on the feet, hands, head and spine as the hands-on approach.

Robert observed that we primarily correspond with life in three ways: thinking, doing and going. He called this the principle of correspondence.

Thus, in order to address all the ways we interact with life, we work on the spinal reflex points for the feet, hands and head.

The spine is the center of the body. The feet, hands and head all extend out from the spine. The spine embodies all that took place during gestation, with the primary focus on the attitudes of mind that created who we are today. These attitudes of mind were created from our genetic and karmic patterns, which entered at conception.

When practicing Metamorphosis, we allow the treatment to take place, just as we allow healing to take place. This means that we do not direct a treatment or aim to heal. To have the intent to heal is a symptomatic approach. When we address the imbalance of afference and efference, healing is the response. (Just a reminder: the word healing is used in this book to mean creating a healthier, happier and more creative approach to life.) I make a point of clarifying this point because Metamorphosis isn't about 'healing.' Metamorphosis is about 'creating' health, harmony, joy...the life that you desire. As a practitioner it is important that you are clear on how these are different intentions.

During the hands-on practice of Metamorphosis, as you place your finger(s) on or above a spinal reflex point, you place your attention there. By placing your attention there, you draw the attention of the recipient's innate intelligence to a block or underlying pattern. I like to use the analogy of holding a flashlight; you are just bringing attention / awareness to a block. It is the recipient's innate/higher intelligence that determines the response.

I like to start a treatment by saying 'hello.' I lightly place my hand on their foot, hand, head or spine, while we both get comfortable with each other. Metamorphosis addresses the core disturbances within a person, so it is nice to establish a rapport first. The treatment proceeds by tuning-in, which allows you to know where to work, how long to work and what kind of pressure or touch you will use, if any. This includes where to start, such as the feet, hands, head or spine, as well as where on the spinal reflex points to begin. There is no way to teach people how to tune-in, other than to suggest that you consciously pay attention to the reflex points until you no longer need to.

You can practice tuning-in by holding a foot and moving your hands along the spinal reflex points, noticing what you feel. You may want to close your eyes if that makes it easier. You will begin to get a sense of where the tension is calling you to begin treatment, without judgment or analysis. As you relax and let your hands or your inner-knowing respond rather than your mind, tuning-in will become natural. It is a matter of trusting your intuition.

The overall theme or intent has already been presented. Now it is time to let that go and simply practice Metamorphosis. Trust that you can do it, you might surprise yourself!

The following pages explain where and how to work.

THE FEET

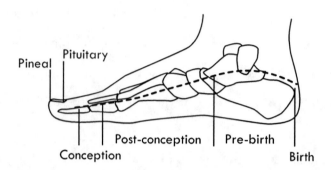

The hands-on approach involves working on the spinal reflex points, which are diagramed above with dotted lines. These dots follow along the bony ridge of the inside edge of the foot.

We work on the feet to address the primary stress patterns. The feet and legs are the extension of the hips, which move us forward in life. The feet

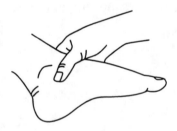

represent the principle of action, our ability or inability to move forward in life.

For the sake of comfort, when working on the area of the big toe, support the toe with your other hand, so as not to stress the joint.

Across the Ankle

The reflex points on the ankle start just below the little round ankle bone on the inside of the foot and continue across the instep, to just below the little round ankle bone on the outside of the foot.

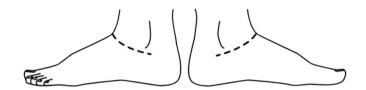

The ankle is considered to be the principle of action. Robert also referred to this area as a 'psychic bustle'. Keep in mind that Metamorphosis is about looking at the principle or nature of things. The ankle is a reflex for the pelvic/hip area, where action or movement is initiated. A bustle is a piece of clothing that you wear around the waist that sits behind you. Robert, in his frequent clever use of words, used the term 'psychic bustle' as an analogy for all the stuff we do not want to deal with, what in a sense, we have shoved out of view.

The action principle represents our ability to move forward. Sometimes we have ideas that we cannot put into motion. Other times we feel 'stuck', as there is a lack of ease in moving through life. When we can't get ideas or ourselves in motion, the action principle may be blocked. This can show physically as problems with the hips, legs, knees, ankles or feet.

You may want to check the ankles prior to working to see how congested they are. I put my hand over the ankle area to get a sense of how it feels. When the action principle is very congested it inhibits the ability to move out of your patterns.

Congestion can feel heavy or chaotic or your hand may feel glued to the spot. If the ankle area feels congested, you may want to begin treatment there. It is advisable to check this area prior to working on someone with a more extreme pattern, such as Down Syndrome. If there is a lot of congestion, you may want to begin the treatment on the ankles and start with shorter treatments.

Characteristics of the Feet

Tissue with tension, due to your underlying stress patterns, has a negative reaction to the stresses imposed on them. He saw this occur regularly with the feet. The rubbing of your shoes on tissue with tension elicits a negative reaction such as bunions, blisters and an array of disorders. It is your underlying patterns, rather than your shoes, that cause the disturbances you experience on your feet.

Consider the nature of these disturbances as to where they physically manifest in relation to the prenatal pattern. Notice the nature of the disturbance: is the area dry, moist, infected or otherwise affected? For example, dryness is a lack of moisture. The moisture is in retreat, so this would be an afferent disturbance.

The characteristics of the disturbances expressed on a person's feet are interesting and often give insight into their story. The disturbances are physical clues as to where some of their underlying stresses lie. Keep in mind this does not mean that you would use this information to determine where or how long to work. We hinder a treatment when we analyze a person or attempt to direct the treatment.

A few examples to get you thinking:

- Blisters are moist bubbles created from friction. Moisture implies emotional tension. The skin is expressing an unhappy reaction to life.

- Calluses create protection, skin building on skin. Look at the nature of where the calluses are. For example, callusing around the heel is associated with birth. Birth represents the principle of action. This may imply a resistance to, or fear of moving forward in life. As a reflex for birth, it could also imply tension in regard to your mother, or your own sense of mothering or nurturing yourself or others.

- Bunions are bone building on bone, which suggests the tension is more deep-seated than skin building on skin. In general, notice where on the foot, in relation to the prenatal pattern, the disturbance lies. A bunion begins to form at the eighth week of gestation. During gestation, the eighth week is when our sense of self is developing. A bunion represents a deep-seated tension in relation to how you feel about yourself. This tension is often unconscious and the person may appear confident.

The Hands

We work on the hands to address the ability to 'do' things or get things done as well as handle life, emotions or a recent Metamorphosis treatment.

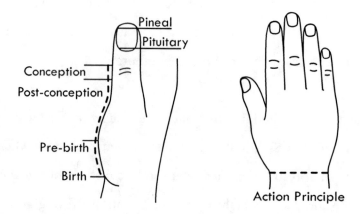

The dotted lines represent the spinal reflex points. As you work down the inner edge of the hand, follow along the bony ridge.

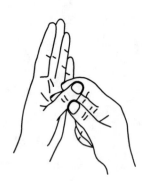

The back of the wrist is the same principle as the ankle. It is the pelvic/ hip reflex, action principle and 'psychic bustle' but in relation to handling and doing things. As with the ankles, you can check the wrists to see how congested they are prior to working on the hands.

For the sake of comfort, support the thumb while working in that area, so as not to stress the joint.

The Head

We work on the head to address the level of tension in relation to thinking. Head or mental tension can create headaches, sinus problems, excessive thinking, worrying, analyzing or mental illness.

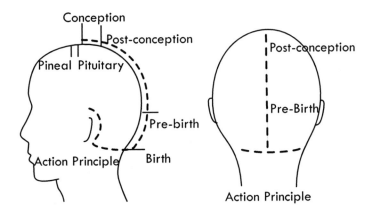

The musculature system reflects the degree of underlying mental tension within a person. Often people cannot relax or stay relaxed, even during or after a massage, because the tension is mental rather than muscular. People with a lot of underlying mental tension often find a Metamorphosis treatment to be surprisingly relaxing.

Working across the base of the skull is similar to working across the ankle or wrist; it is the hip/pelvic reflex and the action principle, but in relation to thinking. Follow the bony ridge along the base of the skull, along the bony ridge behind the ears, to where the top of the ear joins with the head. You can work along one side of the base of the skull and then the other or do both at the same time using two hands. Do what feels most comfortable and appropriate each time.

As with the ankles and wrists, you can check the base of the skull to see how congested it is prior to working on the head. If a lot of congestion is present you may want to begin treatment there. Keep in mind you do not need to work on the ankles, wrist or back of the skull in every treatment. As always, tune-in.

You will want to be mindful with pressure when working on the head, as it is more sensitive than it may appear. Experiment with how pressure feels on your own head.

The Spine

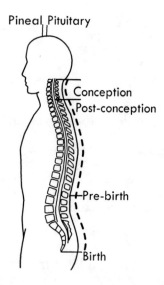

Robert originally said that working on the spine was primarily for animals. Late in life he became more receptive to working on human spines. Basically, he said the spine was too direct of an approach; that working indirectly was more effective, such as working on the spine via spinal reflex points of the feet, hands and head.

While I agree with working as abstractly as possible, I also think that the theme of Metamorphosis itself is as abstract as some people can comprehend at first. I teach working on the spine because I have found benefit from it personally and in working with others. I think of it as providing the degree of structure that some need in order to begin to engage with the principles of Metamorphosis.

Consider the nature of communication. Efference tends to be direct and thus better understands a more direct form of communication. Afference tends to be indirect and thus better understands an indirect form of communication. This is useful in understanding that Metamorphosis is a means to communicate. It is not meant to be used to analyze or diagnose a person or to determine where or how to work.

I encourage you to explore working on the spine and notice the difference in how it feels. Notice the direct nature of working on the spine versus the indirect nature of working on the spinal reflex points on the feet. The spine will probably feel more intense because you are working directly on the prenatal pattern. This is not an indication that it is more powerful, as sensation does not mean a treatment is better or powerful.

You might find you are not inclined to work on the spine, but in doing so, you may gain an awareness of what it means to work with levels of structure. The more abstract you are the less structure you are using.

It does not matter if you work directly on top of the spine, just off to the right or just off to the left, as long as you are making contact with the bony structure. As always, it is the intention that is most important.

You can touch the spine through clothing or directly on bare skin. You can also work away from a clothed or bare spine, just slightly to a few inches above the body.

When working on the coccyx, I tend to work away, just slightly above the coccyx. Most people are not comfortable with touch in that area. I leave my other hand on their low back so they know I am still working, as they cannot see me.

The prenatal pattern on the feet, hands and head are reflex points for the spine. The ankle, wrist and base of the skull are reflex points for the hips. Working on the hips, like the spine, is a more direct form of communication. The hip reflex points begin on the inside edge of the hip crest, across the top of the sacrum and follow along the hip crest to its outer edge. As with the base of the skull, you can work on one hip crest at a time, or both at the same time using two hands. When working on the spine you can check the hips to see how congested the area is prior to starting treatment.

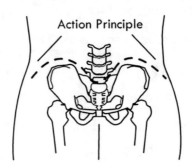

Action Principle

The Spine on Animals

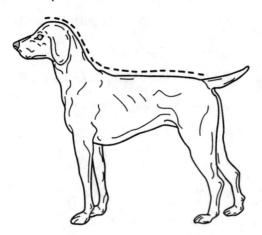

Animals are also subject to the negative relationship between afference and efference.

When working with animals, the same principles and practice apply. Working on the head and spine is more practical than working on paws, claws or hoofs.

Animals do not have the same level of mental tension that humans have and generally respond to a treatment much more quickly. Treatments do not tend to last as long as with humans. Work in the same way as you would with a person, tune-in to know where, how long and how often to work.

After receiving treatments a few times, animals will often let you know, in one way or another, when they are ready for another treatment. They also tend to walk away when they feel the treatment is done.

As with a person, it is important to get permission prior to working on an animal. Animals are usually receptive to telepathic communication. This is done by tuning-in to the animal, presenting your question in thought and quietly waiting for a reply. You do not necessarily hear the reply; you often just know the answer. You can always go by the obvious physical cues. Does the animal sit down and get comfortable or does he walk away from you?

It is possible to be injured by certain animals. I recommend that you gain experience in working with these animals prior to practicing Metamorphosis on them.

Working on Plants

You can work on plants even though they do not have a spine or spinal reflex points. You simply hold the plant stem with the inherent intent to practice Metamorphosis, for as long as it feels appro-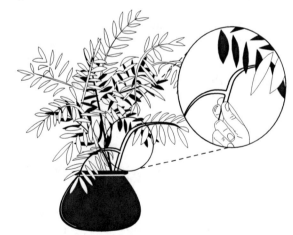
priate. I have actually seen a drooping plant instantly perk up.

Frequently Asked Questions

I have written the remainder of this section in a question and answer format based on the questions I have heard over the years. I listened carefully to all the questions asked. What I heard was a difficulty stepping into a different perspective because people tend to be conditioned with beliefs and ways of thinking. For this reason I chose to address actual questions in this book so that I can clarify the principles.

Please take note of the principles in each response rather than reading them as answers to questions.

Where do I start working?

You will need to tune-in to each person to see whether to start on the feet, hands, head or spine. Metamorphosis is not a technique so there isn't a set way to approach a treatment.

You will also need to tune-in to see where on the foot, hand, head or spine to start working.

It is helpful to realize that you are working with a timeline from conception to birth as well as the movement of awareness into action. Some find it helpful to start at the top, conception /awareness, and work their way down to birth/action.

We are also working, in a sense, with the past and present when working on the feet and hands. The left foot and hand represent what we came into life with. The right foot and hand represent the present. The logic here is that it is helpful to begin working on what is going on in the present. I tend to ask for a foot or hand and start with whichever one is given to me.

Tuning-in and working intuitively is always the way to practice Metamorphosis. I let my hands rather than my mind decide where to start a treatment.

Should I work on the feet, hands, head and spine in every treatment?
Not necessarily. Tune-in to see what feels appropriate in each treatment. Anytime you work without tuning-in, you are operating from technique, which is not as effective. You need to feel what is going on with the person in order to know where to work and for how long.

How long should I work on each foot or hand and the head or spine?
As long as it feels appropriate. It is important that you do not time how long you work on each foot or hand and the head or spine. If you time aspects of the treatment you cannot work intuitively.

One foot or hand may need more attention than the other, which can only be observed by tuning-in. It is typical for the right foot or hand to feel different from the left one, as the left one represents the past and the right one the present.

A treatment may take five minutes or it may take a few hours, depending on what is needed at that time. If time is an issue you can set the intention to have the treatment 'unfold' in a set amount of time, instead of timing each segment.

How long should I stay on each reflex point?
There are different perspectives on this. Some suggest that you do not stay on any one reflex point longer than another, nor do you stay on them for

very long. The idea here is to simply introduce the theme so the other person can respond without your assistance. Staying on a reflex point beyond that is considered to be assisting them.

Others tend to spend more time on reflex points that seem to need it. In practicing the work, I have found that it sometimes takes a while for a person to respond. I also notice that I have spots that seem to need more attention when I receive treatments. I stay on reflex points that seem to need it, often for quite a while. I wait until the sensation I am experiencing eases or until I feel inclined to move my fingers.

Robert saw things in principle. I think sometimes he saw our potential. I also think with the practice of Metamorphosis we naturally move toward the ability to work more abstractly as well as find the ability to create change without assistance. Over time this will sort itself out as we collectively let go of our underlying stresses. Consider these ideas for yourself and see what you think.

When first starting out, I suggest that you stay on each reflex point for longer than you may think you would. This is so that you can develop a sense of tuning-in and notice what blocks feel like. At first you may need to 'go quiet' within yourself as you work on a reflex point and observe what you feel or sense, without analysis. As you begin to embody working intuitively, tuning-in will become second nature and you will not need to consciously pay as much attention.

Eventually, everyone begins to know where to start and end a treatment and how long to stay on a reflex point. It is a matter of just doing it and finding your way with it. No one can teach you how to tune-in, you have to have patience and take a little time to recognize the ability within yourself.

My favorite part about teaching Metamorphosis is seeing people practice on each other for the first time and watching them realize that it works even though they do not understand what they are doing. It is a matter of allowing instead of doing.

Should my fingers move or apply pressure?

At one point Robert suggested that pressure and constant motion were helpful. At another point in time, he started doing a light swirling motion which many have adopted. Some people use a small circular motion as they work along the spinal reflex points.

As you respond to what is being presented to you via the spinal reflex points, you may find that your touch and the amount of pressure you use, if any, changes throughout the treatment.

In general I find it easier to tune-in if my hand is not in constant motion. I let my fingers, rather than my mind, determine if they are going to work on or above the area as well as move or apply pressure, based on what is presented to them as I am working. Respond to the reflex point rather than try to produce change. For some this comes naturally, for others it just takes a bit of time and trust.

Keep in mind that Metamorphosis is not actually bodywork; the focus is not the body. The hands-on approach is a means to introduce the principles and theme of Metamorphosis. How you touch a reflex point is secondary to your intent.

Can I change hands while I am working? Does it matter which hand I use?

Yes, you can change hands, and no, it does not matter which hand you use.

Should I relax someone prior to starting a treatment?

No. The intent of Metamorphosis is to address underlying stress patterns rather than create relaxation. Keep in mind we accept people just as they are. It is okay for tension to be present. However, we do make sure people are comfortable, as we do not want to add tension or discomfort. I provide a pillow for support under the knees if needed and have additional pillows and a blanket available for support or comfort.

How often can a person receive a treatment?

In general not more than once a week, as it can take up to a week for a treatment to finish. Robert used to liken a treatment to cleaning out your cupboards. You start by taking everything out, evaluate what you want to keep or get rid of and put everything back, possibly in a new order. If you have started to put things away and then start to take them all out again, you create chaos. It is usually best to finish what you started before you begin again.

On the other hand, sometimes it feels necessary to receive a treatment more than once a week. Trust your intuition and be mindful of any tendencies to receive treatments too often. We often want to get rid of our discomforts and tend to focus on the symptoms of our patterns. As a result you may work on yourself or receive treatments too often. This can be unsettling as it tends to create chaos, hinders the ability to simply let go of a pattern, and also creates the tendency to work symptomatically.

You can work on your hands to help you handle life and your emotions. Because they are not addressing the primary patterns, you can work on them as often as you feel inclined to. This is helpful in-between treatments.

Do I need to hold the intention of Metamorphosis while I work?

No, the intent is inherent in your decision to practice Metamorphosis. Receiving and giving treatments, reading the literature and considering the philosophy allows you to embody Metamorphosis. The information is there, even if you do not intellectually understand it.

What does a block feel like?

Blocks can feel hot, cold, tingly, chaotic, exhausting upon touch, or it may feel like your hand is glued to the spot. You might experience a physical sensation in your own body while working on someone else. Your arm may feel exhausted or your fingertips may feel hot or cold where they are working. Fortunately, when you are finished, you should no longer experience these sensations. If you do, work on yourself when you can.

Some practitioners have a tendency to over-identify with the patterns of the recipient and can feel a little overwhelmed while working. If you are feeling disturbed as you are working, it is helpful to take a breath or find your own means of coming back to your center.

It is helpful to know that some people do not physically feel blocks, although everyone seems to sense them in one way or another.

How do I protect myself from other people's energy?

It is common in the healing arts to use white light or to ground your energy prior to starting a treatment. Use them if they feel helpful, but keep in mind that if you are in reasonable balance, you won't be negatively affected by the patterns of others.

If someone else's energy is disturbing to you after the treatment is over, then work on yourself. This is actually a nice opportunity for you, as a pattern of your own was obviously stimulated, otherwise their energy would not continue to disturb you.

What should I do if someone starts to emote?
Should I try to elicit emotion for release?

On occasion, a person does experience emotion during a treatment. This is not to be discouraged or encouraged. Let it take place without turning it into a counseling session.

Often in the healing arts the practitioner is encouraged to become involved with a treatment and try to elicit or help someone process emotion. With Metamorphosis we allow rather than assist or elicit. Think about what this means, for it may require a change of perspective for some people.

You can be loving and supportive simply by being present and trusting their innate intelligence, without intervening or interfering.

If you feel inclined, work on their hands, as this helps them to cope with what they are dealing with. I would encourage you to teach them to work on their own hands as well, so that they can continue to work on them at home in-between treatments.

Can I use lotion, oil or powder during a treatment?

You can, but ask yourself, what is the motive? Many years ago, Robert used a healing powder with Metamorphosis. At first he thought this product was in alignment with Metamorphosis. Robert later said the life force or innate intelligence did not need assistance. He realized that using something outside of the self was contradictory to the principles of the work and he no longer encouraged the use of healing products with Metamorphosis.

Can I work on the aura of the foot, hands, head or spine?

Yes, you can. We call it 'working away' from the foot, hand, head or spine. We are actually working on the prenatal pattern and the creation theme in the energy field around the area.

Tune-in to see whether you should work on or away from the skin. Work on yourself to experience how different the two approaches feel.

Can I work on areas other than the spinal reflex points?

You can, but what is your motive? If you are drawn to work somewhere else, then do. The compulsive nature of efference is often compelled to expand and complicate things. It is the simplicity of Metamorphosis that makes it so profound.

Can I work on myself?

Yes! One of the nice things about Metamorphosis is that you can work on yourself. Some encourage solely working on yourself. I prefer to work on myself and also have someone else work on me. Robert used to say that, if possible, it is best to work with someone you have an affinity with, rather than having many people work on you.

Often when you have an affinity with someone you have similar patterns. Whenever you work on someone else, you are in a sense, getting a treatment too. This makes it beneficial to work on family members, as families share similar patterns.

My husband and I work on each other regularly. Keep in mind that a significant other may not be your best choice for a practitioner. Some couples work well as practitioners for each other and other couples do not.

When working on myself, do I have to do a full treatment?

A full treatment is somewhat arbitrary, as a treatment is whatever is needed at the time, which is known by tuning-in. We tend to think in terms of hours, which is a fee-based system.

What if I cannot reach my own feet or spine?

Sometimes it is difficult to reach your own feet. It is fine to use an object, such as the soft eraser at the end of a pencil, as an extension of your hand. For those who appreciate the abstract nature of intention, you can work on your hand and say it is your foot.

It is also hard for most people to reach the full length of their own spine. You can use an object to help you reach the areas you cannot. I use something I found in a health food store called a 'Bonger,' a rubber ball on a flexible metal strip with a comfortable wood handle.

For those who appreciate the abstract nature of intention, you can work on the front of your body with the intention of working directly on the spine. You can also do this in your mind, visualizing a treatment on the feet, hands, head or spine.

Can I work on someone at a distance?

It is preferable to receive a treatment in person. If this is not possible, distance work is a practical option.

Because we are working with intention, you can work on your own foot and say it is someone else's. I find this a little difficult, as I tend to start working on myself. Robert had a plaster model made of his own foot. I found a stuffed bear that has a long body because he is designed to be a foot rest. I use him as a model for the head and spine. You can also work on someone in your mind, visualizing the treatment.

Work in the same way you would work on someone in person, tune-in to the person you are working with to know where and how long to work.

As always, it is important to get permission one way or another. It is tempting to 'fix' or 'help' your friends or relatives by sneaking in treatments, but it is not appropriate. For one thing, you are deciding what is best for them. If a person does not want to change, they won't. If you sneak in a treatment, they may have a reaction to it and not have any reference for what is taking place.

Working on yourself is always the best solution to problems with yourself or others. You may find that the bothersome person is easier to cope with, because you are no longer in reaction to them. As a result, they may even be more receptive to a treatment.

It is nice to know that as you work on yourself, you are indirectly working on those that share your lineage and patterns. As we change, so does the negative dynamic of afference and efference on the planet. Others, including relatives, may change due to you working on yourself.

When working at a distance, can I work on several people at once?

When working at a distance, you are still tuning-in to the individual to know where to work and for how long. It is not possible to effectively tune-in to more than one person at a time.

Am I interfering with a person's life lessons or karma?

The ideas that we have lessons in life, or karma to fulfill, are perspectives or explanations for the problems and challenges in life. The Metamorphosis perspective is that the separation of afference and efference has created humanity's dilemmas. We are subject to the negative relationship of afference and efference, rather than learning lessons.

I think it is helpful to recognize that the person receiving the treatment is making changes within. Change is not imposed; it is a natural result of coming into a better balance of afference and efference. With this in mind, if we are here to learn lessons, I think Metamorphosis will help bring the awareness needed. Lessons don't always have to be hard.

I find it interesting to see how our belief systems shape our reality. Take the time to notice your own beliefs and how they define your purpose, identity and reality. It does not seem possible to be without a perspective on reality, but it is interesting to experience differing points of view and to broaden your possibilities.

How come some treatments seem so 'powerful' and others do not?

People sometimes find a treatment to be very powerful, or rather, full of 'sensation'. Although this is exciting, because you can feel something happening, it does not necessarily mean that it was more beneficial than a treatment that was not 'sensational.'

Sometimes the sensation is due to the practitioner approaching the work in a superficial manner, such as treating symptoms. It is easy to slip into the mode of wanting to help relieve symptoms, but you will not find fundamental or permanent change this way.

What should people expect after a treatment?

Some people fall asleep during and after the treatment. Others feel energized and less tired or stressed, while others do not feel anything at all. Sometimes, as patterns are being worked out, symptoms may seem unusually intense for a few days. Some people feel emotional or out of sorts. In general, it is helpful not to treat symptoms during these times as this may inhibit the Metamorphosis treatment.

I often teach people how to work on their own hands and/or show them the hand symbols. If they do experience difficulties after a treatment they have something they can do about it.

It is helpful to let people know that they may feel tired or emotional during the following week. I like to be clear that these things may happen so that the person does not think the treatment was ineffective or unconsciously create a reaction out of expectation.

Sometimes it feels as if nothing has happened during the treatment. Robert used to say, "when you hit the nail on the head," the pattern is simply gone, without any phenomena. You only remember the problem when you have a reason to recall how you used to be.

How come some people experience strong reactions?

There is no definite explanation for this. It could be that people address their patterns in a similar way in which they approach life. Some people are subtle and others are more dramatic. This could also be an indication that they are receiving treatments too often or that the practitioner is working symptomatically.

Do you have case studies on Metamorphosis?

Robert was against case studies simply because it is necessary to label someone in order to do a study. When you label a person it is harder for them to move out of that pattern, as they have identified with it. This also leads to working symptomatically, because the practitioner is seeking results. When you work symptomatically, symptoms often go away, but they usually return or new ones develop.

Testimonials are a way of showing the diversity of the benefits of practicing Metamorphosis. These are unsolicited observations. When you ask someone to observe their progress they begin to focus on their patterns.

If I am not sure I have the right understanding of the work, will this affect my treatments?

Yes and no. There is a tendency in life to want to be right and do things right. The beauty of Metamorphosis is that there isn't a 'right' way to do it, per se. The key is in understanding the use of intention and the image pattern.

Some people tend to fall into the intellectual trap of thinking they have the right understanding of Metamorphosis. This tends to lock them into a perspective and makes the theme a belief. As a result the work can become dogmatic.

Others hold themselves back from practicing because they are concerned that they do not have the right understanding of Metamorphosis.

Your orientation and patterns influence your understanding. This means that no one has 'the' right understanding unless they are entirely free of stress patterns.

Efference tends to add unnecessary structure and move away from the essence. Afference tends to get caught up in a mental perspective of Metamorphosis and think about the theme, living it more in their minds. This creates an intellectual approach to the work. Fortunately, these things tend to sort themselves out if the person is not too attached to their perspective or orientation.

What I find so exciting about Metamorphosis is that it invites and encourages you to find the answers for yourself. Robert St. John gave us a wonderful structure to work with and an interesting perspective on life, creation and healing. I encourage you to trust yourself enough to find the answers, letting it be okay for your perspective to change. As your patterns shift and change so does your degree of afference and efference. It is natural for your understanding to shift a bit. In the process you will gain a greater understanding of the influence afference and efference have on us.

Is Metamorphosis compatible with other modalities?

Metamorphosis can be compatible with approaches that recognize that we are self-healing. This is sometimes dependent on the orientation of the individual practitioner. The efferently orientated like to follow a structure and tend to direct treatments. The afferently orientated work more intuitively, allowing the innate intelligence to direct the treatment. The efferently orientated trust research and proof. The afferently orientated trust their inner guidance.

The image pattern creates a lot of confusion for people. For this reason I wanted to elaborate on my experience of working with this theme.

The image pattern helps us to see that collectively we have not been using our inner guidance. I think it is important to take this into perspective and not become rigid in your approach. Using assistance from outside of the self isn't wrong. It is helpful to consider this theme and make choices with greater awareness.

To rely only on the self can be the opposite extreme. We live in a dualistic world where all life is connected and yet we are individuals. I appreciate knowing I am supported by a higher consciousness and also appreciate assistance from other people. I have met some insightful teachers over the years that have added to my personal growth. I have also found several healing modalities that helped me along the way. Sometimes I use a supplemental product to support me.

The theme of the Image Pattern has helped me look at the bigger picture. I have become more aware of my choices. What I do is observe. Sometimes I am fearful of my symptoms and look for someone or something to fix me. Sometimes I feel I need assistance with self-healing and other times I feel like I can move through patterns on my own. None of these experiences are right or wrong. I have gained an understanding of the different mind-sets and what happens as a result of stepping into these mind-sets.

Robert had a guardian angel that he frequently talked about. In his seventies he went through a 'healing crisis' where he emerged feeling younger and wiser. During this process his guardian angel became part of him and was no longer outside of himself. In the past he had looked to his guardian angel to help him cope with life's stresses. Now he had more wisdom as well as more responsibility.

Metamorphosis is about taking responsibility and creating greater wisdom or consciousness. Robert's experience occurred naturally with the practice of Metamorphosis. This is the ultimate aim of the work.

Having an awareness of the principles and theme of Metamorphosis helps you move toward them. The practice of Metamorphosis creates this organic process. When we try to 'make' this happen we become dogmatic.

The aim with Metamorphosis is to increase your inner consciousness or awareness. The transition into greater consciousness is challenging. It can feel overwhelming or scary to assume that level of responsibility. It is also quite exciting to realize that you have the ability to make tremendous change within yourself and your life.

I find it is all a journey and every step of it teaches me something. I think it is important to consider the theme of the image pattern and make decisions regarding what you study, practice and receive with greater awareness.

How is Metamorphosis a way of life?

I thought it might be helpful to share how I practice Metamorphosis as a way of life.

I find the principles of Metamorphosis make the most sense and offer their greatest assistance when used during daily life. Metamorphosis is much more than a modality.

When I first learned Metamorphosis it seemed like a huge body of abstract concepts. I felt it was necessary to ground the principles into my daily life so that they could better serve me. Looking at Metamorphosis this way made it easier for me to teach the work, because it made it more understandable and approachable.

I find that observing these principles in daily life allows for the essence of the work to continually reveal itself to me. When you use the principles in daily life they become a part of who you are. This is how you embody the essence of the work and bring the theme to your treatments.

Robert used to say that "you cannot take a person farther than you have gone yourself." While we do not direct a treatment we bring the theme with us. The more we 'know' the theme the better we can impart it during a treatment. When these principles become a part of you, you will also be able to explain the work to others.

Consider how these principles make sense in daily living: motive, identification, blocks and patterns, tuning-in, intention, afference and efference, the image pattern, the use of structure, the practice of Metamorphosis and the theme of creation.

I look at the motives taking place within myself and others. They help me determine how I feel about people. If I know that someone is self-serving I do not spend time with them. If I recognize that they have challenging patterns but their motive is good, I overlook their patterns. If their patterns annoy me, I work on myself.

I notice when people over or under-identify with life, their patterns, an illness, etc. I recognize that it is not helpful to label people or conditions, as this creates limitation.

Tuning-in to the patterns around me on a daily basis has increased my intuition and awareness tremendously. I find that tuning-in to the patterns going on in my daily life helps me to understand the bigger picture. This helps me to move beyond my limitations rather than stay in reaction.

When I tune-in to the dynamic of patterns I don't get as drawn into the drama of life. I tend to take things less personally, using every problem as an opportunity to see my own patterns. I find that once I can see them they tend to get on the move. (This is my own experience and not necessarily the way it should be done. I don't focus on my patterns, I just notice them.)

Recognizing the compulsive nature of patterns within myself has helped me to feel more compassion for other people's patterns. The unconscious and compulsive nature of patterns creates a lot of drama and chaos in life. It is helpful during these times to remember that people don't always realize what they are doing and/or they cannot always help it.

The theme of afference and efference helps my marriage tremendously. Understanding the idea that patterns are unconscious and compulsive along with the relationship pattern has helped my husband and I during our difficult times. We often joke that we would not be married if it wasn't for Metamorphosis.

I find I am more understanding of the people in my life because I recognize the dynamic of afference and efference. I had a very challenging childhood. I am able to come to terms with my past because I can see the bigger picture. It is easier to forgive and move on if you can see the afferent-efferent dynamic and understand that most patterns are unconscious.

I also find that tuning-in to the collective patterns helps me to see why we create the atrocities of life. Looking at the periods of war and suffering throughout history shows me that we really have not moved out of our collective patterns and that work like Metamorphosis is desperately needed. Tuning-in to the nature of war and periods of suffering, such as the current conflict in the Middle East, the Spanish Inquisition or the Holocaust helps me see the extreme negativity in the relationship between afference and efference.

The theme of the image pattern has helped me to take a deeper look at the nature of spirituality and healing.

Recognizing that the scope of the intention determines the scope of the outcome changed how I looked at the healing arts. I can see the limitations and the use of structure in the healing arts. This has helped me to be more discerning in what I choose to work with.

I think spirituality is who we are in our daily living. Taking responsibility for your own patterns and helping to assist others in moving out of their negative patterns, in my opinion, is the ultimate practice of spirituality. As we individually take responsibility and move out of our patterns we will collectively create a more loving and peaceful existence.

Knowing that through the practice of Metamorphosis I am helping to 'save' the planet, create more awareness of animals and the environment, and inspire unconditional love gives my life a greater sense of purpose. This is what inspires me to practice and teach Metamorphosis.

The practice of the work allows me to put the principles to work. I use the creation hand symbol to help me move through the challenges I face in life. I use the hand symbols and practice the hands-on approach throughout the day as needed. My husband and I practice Metamorphosis as our primary approach to dealing with conflict or issues, healing injuries, creating better health, strengthening intuition and manifesting what we want in life.

I see a common theme between trusting the innate intelligence during a treatment as well as during my day-to-day life. I am able to create the life I want when I tune-in to, and trust, my higher self or higher guidance. When I try to create my life from what I think I should be doing things do not go as well. This is allowing versus doing. This is creation, when we are able to create life without effort! This is the ultimate aim of the principles and practice of Metamorphosis.

The principles and practice of Metamorphosis are constants in my life. I find Metamorphosis makes life simple. It provides so much without a lot of structure or effort. I am always inspired by the endless potential of what we can accomplish, when we begin to embody the principles and practice of Metamorphosis as a way of life!

Why are there different perspectives on the teaching and practice of Metamorphosis?

There are several reasons for this. Robert spent his life writing about, working with, and refining the theme of Metamorphosis. He regarded his writings as a means to see the progression of thought more than a collection of data. His focus was on developing the work and he did not go back and edit his books.

This meant one needed to have fairly frequent contact with him to hear his latest insights.

Robert wrote about the prenatal pattern in his book *Metamorphosis, a Text Book on Prenatal Therapy* and about afference and efference in his *Introductory Articles*. You will find people working with Metamorphosis from varying perspectives, depending on when they were introduced to the work, who they studied with and what book(s) they have read. Their afferent or efferent orientation will also influence how they approach the work.

Robert's early work, Prenatal Therapy, evolved into Metamorphosis when he began including afference and efference and the image pattern into his perspective.

Because Metamorphosis is a philosophy and not a technique, it allows for people to teach from their own understanding. This enables people to embody the theme, practicing and teaching from an inner understanding. This means that there is more variation in how people teach the work, which sometimes creates confusion for students who study with different people.

~ ~ ~

I find it is helpful to engage with the essence and not get too bogged down with the data of the work. Remember, the data is simply a blueprint that allows you to 'step into' the theme of Metamorphosis. It is important to have an awareness of the principles and theme but it is not necessary to intellectualize them.

We are innately self-healing and are capable of creating a healthier and more positive approach to life. All you need to do is remember that and step out of the way. Have fun with it. Allow the understanding to come to you rather than trying to intellectually understand Metamorphosis, life or healing.

The less you 'think' about how to work the better. The hands-on approach is subject to your intention and motive, rather than technique. If you know where the spinal reflex points are and have a sense of the principles, you are ready to go. The work really is simple if you seek its essence, enjoy!

TREATMENT LOCATION

The most important consideration when deciding where to give a treatment is that you are both comfortable. Metamorphosis is a practical approach to healing. A special healing environment, while nice, is rarely practical in daily living and by no means necessary.

A sofa is a comfortable place to work on the feet and hands. As the practitioner, you sit facing forward and the recipient sits or lies comfortably with

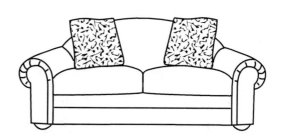

their foot or hand in your lap. You may want to put a small pillow or towel on your lap, and a pillow under their extended knee for support.

You can also work sitting in chairs. Place the chairs at 90-degree angles, which will look like an L shape. When working on the feet, put your knee under their extended knee so that it is supported rather then stressed.

Robert used to say he preferred to work on a sofa or in chairs. Sitting at relatively the same eye level creates a sense of equality. When someone lies down on a massage table, they have the inherent mind-set to be 'healed by' another. The positioning is un-equal and has the connotation that the practitioner is a healer or an authority.

Even though I agree with Robert, I use a massage table when I work on the spine. I find the face cradle on the massage table is convenient for working on the head and spine, as the recipient does not have to strain their neck by turning their head to one side. This also allows me to be able to sit or stand comfortably.

I would not recommend buying a massage table just to practice Metamorphosis. It is practical for working on the spine and head, but not necessary. If you are working on friends and family, be creative and use a bed or futon. I have seen body support cushions in catalogues. If so inclined, you will find something that will work.

It is possible to work on a person's head while they are sitting in a chair. This works best if the practitioner is standing behind the recipient. It is helpful to support the person's head by putting one hand on their forehead, allowing the weight of their head to fall into your hand. You can also work on the spine with the recipient turned to face the back of a chair, with their spine facing you. Use pillows in front so that it is comfortable to lean into the back of the chair. My husband and I often work on each other's head and spine while lying in bed.

A Few Things to Consider When Working with Others

If you decide that you would like to practice Metamorphosis in a professional manner, please remember that you need to work in accordance with the laws in your area. Some places require a license to touch, such as massage certification or a Minister's license.

Listed below are a few situations you may want to consider. Some situations, such as pregnancy, have additional benefits, while other situations may warrant consideration on your part. This is not to deter you from working with anyone. If someone asks for, or wants to receive a treatment, trust that he knows what is best for himself. What I am trying to impart here is that you need to be comfortable as a practitioner to follow through with treatments once they are started.

Pregnancy / Pregnant Women

Working with pregnant women is helpful to both the mother and baby. The mother's underlying patterns are being addressed, which will help her to be a healthier and more relaxed parent. The patterns of the baby are also being addressed, which will allow the baby to move through the developmental stages with less tension and resistance. Babies that receive treatments while in the womb are born with less underlying tension, which will make their lives easier from the beginning.

Metamorphosis treatments during pregnancy often result in a shorter, easier labor as well. This is due partly because the tension in the pelvic region of the mother has been addressed and primarily because the baby, after receiving treatments, is more able and willing, or less resistant, to coming forward into life.

You will want to be mindful of working on the ankle (action principle) during pregnancy so as not to over-stimulate the area and inspire labor to begin.

To work on a pregnant woman's spine, she may need to lie on her side with pillows between her legs and knees for support. Ask her where else she may need additional support from a pillow or rolled up blanket or towel.

The Elderly

The elderly are often preparing to pass on. Remember, you do not determine what takes place; the person receiving the treatment does. If the person does choose to depart, they most likely will do so with less stress or tension. Metamorphosis treatments may help with their transition.

Children

Children do not usually have the degree of mental tension that most adults do. Because of this, treatments do not always take as long as with an adult. Children usually know when the treatment is finished and often get up and walk away. You may also find their feet in your lap, as they usually know when they need another treatment.

It is helpful to work on as many willing family members or caregivers as possible, especially if the home environment is abusive or unhealthy. Due to family dynamics, one or more relatives often resent the person who is changing. Some parents just want you to 'fix the problem,' which is how they often view the child. The parents may not be open to considering that they may be part of the situation.

Children do not have the freedom to move on to healthier surroundings as their own patterns shift. To get a glimpse of a better life and not be able to obtain it can be disheartening. On the other hand, they may be better able to cope with their environment. How does the child feel about receiving treatments? If at all possible, you can teach the child how to work on himself, so that he has a means to help himself.

People in Confined Locations

People in confined locations have a similar situation to children, as they are not always free to move to a healthier environment. People in a mental hospital are a good example. After receiving treatments, they may begin to find their way out of their inner dilemma, but still be subject to forced medication and confinement. They may get a glimpse of a better means of functioning, but not be able to obtain it.

On the other hand, the individual may find it easier to cope with their environment and possibly find a way out of their situation.

Some people are temporarily confined, such as a person serving time in prison. Upon release, they may find it easier to integrate back into society after receiving treatments.

Animals

Animals tend to be very receptive to Metamorphosis and seem to know what it is you are presenting to them. I have a cute story of a cat and a little dog I met one day while standing on someone's porch. As I am partial to cats I started to work on the cat. The dog began jumping up and down at my feet. Telepathically I heard him say, "work on me." At the same time I heard the cat say, "work on the dog." I told the woman who lived with them what I had heard and she said, "Oh, the dog has cancer and the cat really likes the dog." It was apparent by both of their reactions that they comprehended the act of extending my hand in offer of Metamorphosis.

Keep in mind that not all animals have the freedom to do as they please. The consciousness expressed toward animals is often inhumane. Animals can have a situation similar to children and people in confined locations. You may want to consider the nature of the animal's situation. Some animals are confined to a cage. Other animals are owned and used for labor or are trained for a particular purpose. They basically render themselves to the will of their owner or trainer, often out of fear.

Metamorphosis un-conditions the mind, which means as their independence of mind returns, they may lose or disregard any training they may have received. To find that independence of mind and then be re-trained back into submission can be very disheartening.

In some instances you may want to suggest working with the 'owner' as well, as the negative pattern of afference and efference plays out between all forms of life.

Autism

As with any situation, look at the nature of the pattern, rather than label the person with a condition. Autism is an extreme afferent pattern, a compulsive, chronic retreat from life. Those considered to be autistic, while very intelligent, are overwhelmed by the efference of life, including touch, noise or even direct eye contact.

It is important to be very respectful of their afference. Tune-in to your own afference, approaching them slowly while making indirect eye contact. Make sure they are comfortable with you prior to suggesting that you work on their feet or prior to reaching for them. Respect any decision to refuse a treatment and possibly try again at a later time.

Of course, with anyone, you need to get their permission. Permission can be given verbally, psychically if they are unable to speak, or physically. For example, do they willingly give you their foot or do they pull it away? I would not recommend working on their spine as this would be too direct for them.

Down Syndrome

Again, look at the nature of the pattern. Those considered to be Down Syndrome are easy to recognize as their facial features are often pushed 'outwards.' This is an extreme efferent pattern.

While working with Down Syndrome babies, Robert found that it is possible to actually move out of this pattern. He noticed that even their facial features changed after receiving Metamorphosis treatments during infancy.

Robert observed that the greatest opportunity for change with this pattern occurred within the first five years of life. This is not to suggest that treatments are not beneficial later in life, but they are not as dramatic.

People often ask if there is a special way to work on people with Down Syndrome. You may want to be gentle in your manner, but as with everyone, tune-in and work for as long as it feels appropriate. Check the area around the ankle. If you feel a lot of activity or exhaustion there, you may want to start working on the ankles and/or work for a short period of time.

THE HAND SYMBOLS

The hand symbols are a more abstract approach to working with the same principles and theme as the hands-on approach.

In relation to the level of structure, the hand symbols are more abstract and therefore a more afferent approach to the theme of Metamorphosis.

Whereas the hands-on approach is more direct and therefore a more efferent approach. Within the hands-on approach the spine is more direct than the feet.

Of the six hand symbols, four address aspects of pre-conception, the karmic patterns prior to physicality. Keep in mind we use the word karmic to mean 'of the past' and in the realm of thought. This differs from the Hindu perspective on karma.

One hand symbol addresses conception, the moment in time when all the genetic and karmic influences come together into physical form and one addresses the balance of afference and efference.

While holding the hand symbols, you can place your hands in your lap, or if lying down, on your chest or stomach, whatever is comfortable.

Please note that the hand symbols are used primarily for working on yourself. You can teach a client how to use them at home in between treatments but they are not meant to be used on a client during a treatment.

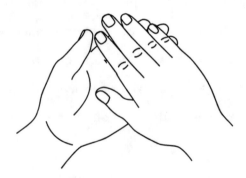

Pineal
Fingers crossing at right angles to each other.
It does not matter which hand is placed on top or how your thumbs are placed.

The pineal gland is the first point that registers the non-material aspects of who we will become.

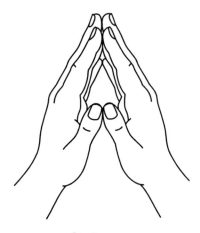

Pituitary
Tips of the fingers and thumbs are touching.

This is the symbol for the pituitary gland, where the genetic patterns of past

generations are introduced and interpreted.

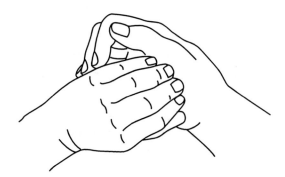

Cupped Hands
One hand cupped over the other.
It does not matter which hand is on top.

This symbol represents our personal or direct karmic patterns.

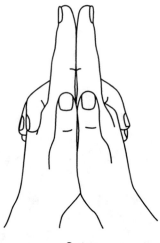

Spire
*All fingers clasped together, except the index fingers, which
are extended upward while touching each other. The outside edges
of the thumbs touch each other as well.*

This symbol represents our indirect karmic patterns.

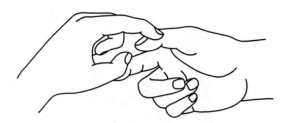

Conception
*The index finger of one hand is touching the conception point
on the opposite hand. The conception points are
the thumb joints on the inside edge of the hand.*

This hand symbol symbolizes the moment of conception, the moment in
time when your genetic and karmic patterns enter into physical form, and
condition the first cell. The conception hand symbol looks a bit tricky at first,
but it is just holding the conception points on each thumb, with a finger of
the opposite hand.

Place your right index finger on the conception point on the left hand. Then swivel the left index finger around and place it on the conception point of the right hand. You can relax your hands while keeping the fingers on the conception points on each thumb.

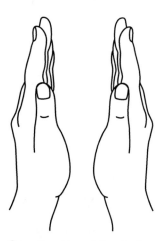

Creation Hand Symbol
Open, flat hands parallel to each other, not touching.

This symbol represents the principle of oneness, enabling you to find a temporary balance of afference and efference. This symbol is helpful to use whenever you feel out of sorts in any way.

You can sit comfortably with your hands in your lap, or if lying down, on your chest. The distance between them is not important. Place your hands where they feel comfortable.

FREQUENTLY ASKED QUESTIONS

How will I know which hand symbols to use?

Familiarize yourself with how to hold the hand symbols, rather than remember what they mean. That way, you will use the one(s) that you feel inclined to use, rather than one(s) you think you should.

To get familiar with the hand symbols, take some time holding each one, noticing how they feel to you. You may get a sense of which one(s) you feel inclined to work with, which often changes over time.

How long should I hold the hand symbols?

There is no set time limit for holding a hand symbol. Hold them as long as it feels appropriate, from a second to a few hours.

How often can I use them?

As often as you feel inclined to use them. Be mindful of any compulsive tendencies to work on yourself too often.

How many should I use?

There is no formula for using them, use as few or as many as you feel inclined to.

Can I use just the hand symbols instead of the hands-on approach?

Yes, if you feel inclined to. Later in his life, Robert primarily used the hand symbols. Using the creation hand symbol, sometimes for hours at a time, he shifted out of his arthritic pattern. He called this his "Grand Morph."

This is the healing crisis I referred to when Robert's guardian angel became part of him.

What if I cannot hold them just right?

Hold them the best you can, while still being comfortable. As always, the inherent intent of Metamorphosis is of primary importance. How you hold the hand symbol is of secondary importance.

Can I use the hand symbols to practice Metamorphosis at a distance?

Yes, you can use them to work on people or animals at a distance, with their permission of course. Simply hold the hand symbol with the intent that it is for a particular person.

Can I use the hand symbols to help with a situation?

Yes, but consider your motive? People often use the creation hand symbol when addressing a situation. It is best to work on the aspect of yourself that is involved with a negative situation rather than directing it at other people.

The situation usually resolves itself once you move out of, or change, an aspect of the pattern that attracted the situation to you.

Can I use hand symbols in meditation?

The hand symbols are not designed to be used in meditation. People usually meditate to bring about a particular state of mind. The hand symbols are a more abstract way to address our underlying patterns.

There is no benefit to structuring the use of the hand symbols, such as using them during a meditation. This would be using them as a technique and would alter the motive for using them.

While working with the hand symbols is a more abstract approach, the principles of Metamorphosis remain the same.

~ ~ ~

I HOPE YOU ENJOY THE JOURNEY!

Suffix to the Functional Human

By Robert St. John ©

(Robert wrote an article called *The Triangle* which he re-named *The Functional Human.* This suffix offers a timeline of shifts with afference and efference. The article can be found in it's entirety in his book *Introductory Articles.*)

For many millions of years this planet has suffered an unrelieved pattern of stress in the form of the potential strain between the two primary elements in life—afference and efference. In all of historical time there have been prophesies concerning "the end of the world," the Armageddon and numerous other warnings of the end, if we go on with the existing methods of living.

In my observation of the polarity patterns of humans I was able to observe a fundamental change which took place in February of 1962. It was a change that indicated a different relationship of afference and efference and a prospect for the future.

There was another change in 1988, and again, another in 1991. A final change has taken place recently (1993). In each of these changes there were very definite indications in the behavior of people that something was 'going on.'

In the first of these three changes the indication was of a change in the way humans were taking their responsibility for their life; it was a change from a reference to an outside source to their own inner self.

The second indication showed a change in the energy content of afference. This began to alter the capacity of afference to 'activate' efference. It had a very disturbing effect on efference.

The third change was that afference and efference were both fully activated, creating an even more disturbing effect on the behavior of the human.

The final change is the most surprising—afference and efference have changed places—they have returned to their original positions of the time before this planet was created. But there is still a duality.

Metamorphosis Certification

Robert St. John chose not to create certification for practicing or teaching Metamorphosis. Metamorphosis is about breaking down the structure of hierarchy, reminding people that we can all create change from within and that we can set this in motion ourselves. The structure of certification creates a level of authority, and requires you to look to a governing body, which takes away from the primary intent of the philosophy.

Metamorphosis is about taking responsibility for your patterns and creating change from within. The responsibility is also on you to respect the nature of what Metamorphosis is about, creating a fundamental change in the relationship of afference and efference, and moving out of the image pattern.

If you decide you like aspects of Metamorphosis but want to mix it with other things or delete aspects of its philosophy, it is no longer Metamorphosis because you have changed its primary intent. It is helpful if you say that the work you are doing is based on aspects of Metamorphosis. That way you do not mislead people or alter someone else's work.

People often recognize the importance of this work and want to teach it. Keep in mind that it is necessary to embody the principles, so that your teaching comes from within. Metamorphosis takes time to integrate into your awareness. It is important to take the time to understand the image pattern, so that you do not inadvertently bring Metamorphosis into the image pattern, thus defeating its purpose.

The responsibility is placed on you, as there are no governing bodies for Metamorphosis, thus the transition into the Aquarian, when people will begin to take responsibility and truly think for themselves.

About the Author

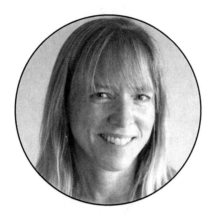

Cindy's passion is to provide support in helping others connect to the magic of working with intention. Teaching Metamorphosis is one of her greatest joys! She has been teaching Metamorphosis classes since 1991. Her background includes a B.A. in Psychology, training in hypnotherapy, massage, Reiki and various alternative modalities.

Cindy studied Metamorphosis with Lynn Hatswell and Robert St. John in Perth, Australia in 1989. She sponsored a lecture for St. John in California and several lectures with international speakers. She also created the U.S. Metamorphosis Journal in 1995 for St. John to inform us of his new developments. The journal was in print through 2001, when Cindy decided to use her energy to write this book.

Cindy is available to lecture and teach. Please contact her if you would like to sponsor a lecture or class in your area or country.

Resources

www.MetamorphosisCenter.com

This web site serves as a resource for Metamorphosis.
Books
Classes
Articles
International Directory of Practitioners

For more information please contact:
The Metamorphosis Center
Cindy Silverlock
PO Box 2945
Santa Rosa, CA 95405 USA

Email: cs@metamorphosiscenter.com

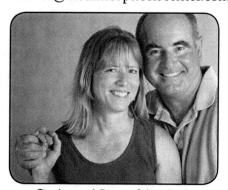

Cindy and Dean Silverlock

Printed in the United States
112592LV00002B/9/P

9 780972 289740